AF730617

THE

WEIGHT MANAGEMENT

DIARY

MIRELLE VRAIMONT

THE WEIGHT MANAGEMENT DIARY

The food groups and combinations are not intended as a cure for anything and should not be regarded as such. The author/publisher confirms the originality of the information presented and the manufacturer is neither liable nor obligated to authenticate, research, or correct.

The views expressed in this book do not reflect the views of the manufacturer or members of the manufacturing staff. These views are solely inured to the author/publisher. The views expressed by the author/publisher in this book are NOT a cure for any pre-existing condition; are NOT to be considered a deterrent to any condition; and are NOT meant as replacement for advice coming from your primary care physician/specialist.

Manufactured in the United States of America by www.lulu.com
ISBN: 978-0-6151-3537-3

DEDICATION

To my children:

Ehrika Aileen Carter Gladden
Jessica Faye Carter
David George Carter, Jr.
Blayne Anthony Gladden
Jennifer Mary Gallagher Carter

The longer I live, the more I believe, there is nothing I have accomplished that is greater than the countless hours I have spent with you and the many things we have shared as you have accomplished your goals.

Your talents were many, your disappointments manageable, your attitudes healthy, and your achievements admirable.

Here's wishing you years of unbridled happiness and love!

Has anyone ever said to you,

EAT WHAT YOU WANT AND BE THE SIZE YOU WANT TO BE NATURALLY!

Well, I hope so because your weight *can* be managed but **ONLY YOU** can manage your weight. Only you are there 24/7, 365/6 and, therefore, only your have absolute control. No doctor, diet guru, nutrition specialist, food counselor, or health counselor can say definitively, 'This is what you should eat for optimum health." They can say "fresh foods are good for you; fresh foods steamed and baked are generally more healthful than fried." They can tell you which oils have less saturated fats and trans-fatty acids. They can delineate aerobic and stretching exercises that can be used to great advantage. However, biochemical individuality, food sensitivities (violent or benign), previous illnesses, prior medications, present medications, blood type, genetics, caloric intake and other factors can cause negative reactions. This guide will help **YOU** manage **YOU!**

If you have not been used to managing your caloric intake—Excellent! You will need to do this through approximately 30 four-day cycles, weighing yourself after each four days. Imagine, after four months, you will know exactly what **YOUR** body will and will not respond to and tolerate; what things negatively impinge on your weight; what things affect your physical health; how to maintain **YOUR** weight. That puts you in total control of your weight forever.

In this weight management diary, you will put in the foods you like. You will choose what and where you want to eat. You will choose reasonable portions. You will, through the suggestion list, be introduced to foods of which you may not have heard. You will learn to count all foods. You will be able to eat everything you love, unless you determine that it is causing you to hold water, swell, etc. When you have completed this you will have not only control of your weight, but a way to keep it in total control and further manage any dietary indiscretions, which we *all* will have from time to time.

If weight is a concern for you, by now you have probably used every diet marketed to alleviate the poundage that creeps up as a result of (in our usual set of excuses) age, eating like a "bird," low will power, emotional eating, anti-cancer medication, hormones, thyroid troubles, weak bones, glandular disturbances, over-sugared and over-salted foods, poor quality food chain, lack of essential fatty acids, etc. When we have tried these diets, we only have the pounds return time and again and often after strenuous "will power" tactics to keep in off. It is important to remember that weight management is not an easy task but your weight can be managed.

America is in for the fight of its life! Obesity has reached epidemic proportions and threatens the life, health, welfare, and well-being of more than two-thirds of the population, young and old. We have survived from time immemorial and will continue to do so, but at what weight?

Inevitably, after much "ado" about taking off the weight, exercising strenuously; lifting weights; counting endless calories; sugars; sodium; fats; "carbs" ad nauseaum; you only see the scales continue to rise. In the typical fashion you beat your self up for having regained the pounds lost through much effort and the cycle begins again!

When looking at the reasons stated above, you may be able to attest to one or more of them being true in your particular "battle of the bulge." However, let's take the ones that are the most applicable to a generality of situations and see what the outcome is!

What are we to do as the children get larger by the hour, lazier by the minute, and hungrier by the second? Of course, as always, there is the talk of behavioral modification, eating less, thinking differently about food, substituting activities (for eating), remembering your vitamins, paying attention to what you like, drinking less alcohol, exercising more, smoking less, making love more, finding a hobby, etc. Remember these? How about this one: **"YOU ARE WHAT YOU EAT!"**

One thing is certain! We are all biochemically individual and that individuality is affected by everything we put in our mouths. Salt swells one person and doesn't affect another. Corn causes one to hold water and does not affect another. Sugar causes one to gain three pounds at one sitting and another is totally unaffected. Here is a statement that most of us are unwilling to admit to**: EVERYONE WHO IS OVERWEIGHT-- SLIGHTLY, CHRONICALLY, OR MORBIDLY (with no medical diagnosis to the contrary)—EATS TOO MUCH AND EXERCISES INSUFFICIENTLY!**

While it may be difficult to admit, if one keeps a running diary of what one eats, when it is eaten, etc., one would find that dietary indiscretions are almost always to blame for weight gain. It is difficult to be in total control of everything that we put in our mouths so the Weight Management Diary will allow you to look at yourself in the mirror and say, I am five pounds overweight and I know why: "Last Monday, I ate an extra bowl of ice cream, Wednesday, I had a whole bag of potato chips, Thursday I had two servings of lobster bisque, and crème brulee for dessert on Sunday."

The trick here is to determine what puts weight on *your* body and decline that particular substance or eat it and then compensate through less calories or more exercise. This can be compensated for when you have a less stressful day.

You can give your self the mindset to complete this short four-month run by asking yourself the following questions and answering them truthfully!

1. Do I eat too much?

2. Do I need all the food I eat to sustain me in the course of the day?

3. Do I know how much I have eaten or do I eat heartily and then claim not to know why I have gained?

4. Do I always eat until I can feel my food "hang heavy?"

5. Do I eat to the point of discomfort?

6. Do I diet incessantly?

7. Do I show any signs of an eating disorder?

8. Do I use eating, snacking, etc., as a substitute when I have no other activities?

9. Do I have closets and closets of clothes I cannot wear?

10. Do I have a sweet tooth?

11. Do I have undiagnosed food allergies (this will be discussed later)?

12. Do I have specific food textures/tastes I must consume or I will feel totally deprived? For example, crispy, creamy, bitter, tart, tangy, salty, sweet, etc.

13. As a vegetarian, isn't it necessary to have a range of tastes?

14. Do I measure the effects of food on me or do I eat and have no idea how I am being affected unless it is a particularly violent reaction?

15. Do I take prescription/otc medicines to control gastric distress related to overeating/drinking?

16. Do I have any internal (mind) controls over what I put in my mouth?

17. Am I in charge of what I eat or is my body?

18. Do I think it is unnecessary to take vitamins because food has all the vitamins I need?

19. Am I a bread fanatic? Why?

20. Do I believe I am making all the dietary adjustments I need to make by using "lite," "lowfat," "diet," etc., as necessary "food types" to help me lose weight?

21. Is most of the food I eat to feed my body or is it emotional compensation, tied to some past psychological event in my life?

22. Do I believe that diet pills or loss of weight by surgical assistance is a necessity?

23. Is my food stimulating?

24. Do I seek stimulation totally from food or do I have the ability to be stimulated through other activities.

25. If my child rejects food, do I demand he/she "clean the plate?" (You can choose this opportunity to give your child a lot of fresh foods and allow his/her self-limitations to develop. Cleaning or not cleaning the plate does not make any hungry child around the world less hungry!)

26. Do I understand that eating what I want and eating well can be a prescription for maintaining an acceptable weight?

If you answer yes to any three of these questions, please consider the following. This book wants you to do six things before you eat: (1) Think differently about what you put in your mouth and count it (calorically); (2) Remember to take your vitamins; (3) Pay attention to the things you like and determine if they "like" you; (4) Read the blood type literature and decide what foods you should be eating for health, which ones you can get away with eating and which ones are poison to your particular blood type, (5) Exercise often, and (6) With every bite/swallow you take, "**OPT FOR HEALTH!"**

Also, consider these statements with respect to their applicability to your situation/health/personal preferences, etc.

1. Remember your vitamins (with our food chain in the condition it is in, think of taking vitamins as insurance).

2. Smoking is detrimental to most people's health.

3. Excessive drinking is detrimental to most people's health.

4. It is important to be able to count what you put in your mouth because if you can't you have no idea how much you are eating.

5. Exercise is important to the cardiovascular, bone, and muscular health of most people. Stretching is equally important for the release of sugar from the muscles and may be more pleasant for some temperaments.

6. The fresher the food the better the opportunity to take in live substances that are life giving. (The so-called debate regarding fresh vs. processed does not exist. It can be quelled with one statement: "Life begets life.")

The first two four-day cycles will be suggested for you with the ability to adjust according to your personal preferences. Information will also be provided for vegan/vegetarians. (If you are a lacto-ovo vegetarian or vegan you can adjust any and all choices to your preferences. By now, your repertoire is extensive for supplementing in the major food groups.)

You may then repeat the two four-day cycles or select and substitute your own foods for the subsequent days until you reach your goal. Remember, if you do not have these foods in the house, substitute a food group equivalent: carbohydrates, proteins, fruits, grains, legumes, dairy, etc. After you have reached your goal, you will remember the things that worked best for you and you will find that you can use this Weight Management Diary to keep or put you right back on track. It is always at your fingertips.

And remember: **EVERYONE WHO IS OVERWEIGHT,-- SLIGHTLY, CHRONICALLY, OR MORBIDLY (with no medical diagnosis to the contrary)—EATS TOO MUCH AND EXERCISES INSUFFICIENTLY!**

1. Five snacks are listed for each day. Have all, any, or none.

2. Buy juices unsweetened, i.e., only with their naturally occurring sugars; canned fruits packed in their own juice.

3. We have all been fighting the weight problem long enough to know that food preparation is very important. Think of it this way: "I love fried chicken. I can have it once a month. I probably shouldn't have it *every* time I eat chicken."

4. Vegetables should be prepared in the shortest time possible. Steamed, baked, sweated, etc. Servings should be limited to ¾ cup.

5. The use of sweeteners is preferred if they don't "swell your head." That is a phrase I use to say that after eating something, it doesn't seem to agree with **ME**. Try any three or four of the popular market brands to see if they agree with you. Also remember the natural one from Brazil, stevia.

6. Use sugar and butter if you want. Butter always, sugar sparingly, as the word is not in on its possible contribution to the diabetes epidemic.

7. Coffee and tea in moderation. If you have one at breakfast, try the other at lunch/snack. Try some of the herbal brands also, but whatever you take in, be aware of how it affects **YOUR** body.

8. When considering your cereals, do you do better with rice, wheat, or oats? Do some of these cause insulin insufficiency? Are you tired and sleepy after using them? If so you may need to consider quinoa, spelt, buckwheat, amaranth, etc., (other grains that can be purchased) from you local health food store.

9, Salt is not forbidden unless you have hypertension or other contraindications for sodium use.

10. **FREELY SUBSTITUTE ANY FOOD ON THE SUGGESTED LISTS BUT DO TRY TO MATCH CARB FOR CARB, PROTEIN FOR PROTEIN, FRUIT FOR FRUIT, ETC., ACCORDING TO YOUR *PERSONAL PREFERENCES*.**

11. Use black, navy, white, pinto, pink, kidney or any other beans and lentils as a free ½ cup snack every third day while following this weight management plan.

12. To address the male/female loss patterns: Men-You may add 2-4 ozs. of meat to your servings (protein) and can feel free to eat all the snacks with few restrictions. Women should take the lowest ounce recommendation and avoid beans/lentils except on an eight-day recurrence. These specifications are made for women because of the hormonal interruption to female metabolism.

DISCLAIMER: WHEN YOU ARE UNDERTAKING ANY WEIGHT LOSS PROGRAM, DO NOT BEGIN WITHOUT THE CONSENT OF YOUR PRIMARY CARE/SPECIALTY PHYSICIAN. USE GOOD JUDGMENT AND NEVER UNDERTAKE ANY PROGRAM CONTRARY TO YOUR WELL BEING PARTICULARLY IF YOU SUFFER FROM OTHER MALADIES AND TAKE PRESCRIBED MEDICATIONS. NO RECOMMENDATIONS MADE IN THIS BOOK MAKE CLAIMS FOR CURES; THE LISTS ARE MERELY COMPOSED OF THE BASIC FOOD GROUPS IN THEIR MOST NATURAL FORM COMBINED IN A VARIETY OF WAYS.

Cycle 1 (4 days)

Substitutions/notes/symptoms Indiscretions/distress/extra calories/etc.

____
____
____
____

Exercise	Duration

Total calories burned______

HOW DO I FEEL TODAY? WAS THERE SOMETHING I ATE THAT DID NOT AGREE WITH ME?

Monday	Breakfast	Lunch	Dinner
	2 eggs	6 ozs. Chicken Salad	4 ozs. Pork
	1 slice toast	1 green salad	1 cup string beans
	1 pat butter	1 cup celery/carrot juice	½ cup coleslaw
	1 pineapple juice	1 cup canned pears/or raw	1 cup buttered rice
	1 coffee/tea	1 coffee/tea	Cranberry juice

Snacks

1 Apple
½ cup peaches
1 ½ ozs. black walnuts
1 herbal tea

*Vegans replace dairy products with soy cheese and reconstituted non dairy creamer. Every third day all weight managers should eat 1/2 cup beans, lentils, and other legumes.

**Vegans/Vegetarians replace meat products with "chicken" (mushroom) tenders and meatballs (mushrooms). Full range of Quorn ® products is suggested for variety. You may also use soy products for protein intake if not a cancer survivor.

Substitutions/notes/symptoms Indiscretions/distress/extra calories/etc. __________ __________ __________ __________ **Exercise Duration** **Total calories burned______**

REMEMBER TO TAKE YOUR INDIVIDUALLY PLANNED SUPPLEMENTS EACH DAY

Tuesday	Breakfast	Lunch	Dinner
	1 ½ ounce cereal *4 ozs. milk 1 cup canned peaches 1 English muffin W/all fruit spread Coffee/tea	**6 ozs. Tuna salad w/ toast Spinach Salad Fruit cocktail Elderberry juice Coffee/tea	**4 ozs. Beef Asparagus Rice pasta Parsnips

Snacks

Veggie chips
8 ozs. kefir
4 tbsps. peanuts
1 herbal tea

***Vegans replace dairy products with soy cheese and reconstituted non-dairy creamer. Every third day all weight managers should eat 1/2 cup beans, lentils, and other legumes.**

**** Vegans/Vegetarians replace meat products with "chicken" (mushroom) tenders and meatballs (mushrooms). Full range of Quorn ® products is suggested for variety. You may also use soy products for protein intake if not a cancer survivor.**

Substitutions/notes/symptoms Indiscretions/distress/extra calories/etc.

____

____

____

____

Exercise Duration

Total calories burned______

COUNT WHAT YOU PUT IN YOUR MOUTH. YOU'LL BE GLAD YOU DID!

Wednesday	Breakfast	Lunch	Dinner
	egg beaters® omelet scrambled with peppers/ onions /topped:sour cream	Turkey Salad	4-6 ozs. fish
	1 slice toast w/butter	Green salad	Zucchini
	Coffee/tea	½ cup pineapple	Carrots
		Coffee/tea	½ cup buttered pasta
		Raw carrot juice	

Snacks

1 oz. potato chips
8 elderberry juice
½ cup canned/fresh apricots
1 herbal tea

***Vegans replace dairy products with soy cheese and non-dairy creamer reconstituted.**

****Replace meat products with "chicken" (mushroom) tenders and meatballs (mushrooms). Full range of Quorn ® products is suggested for variety. You may also use soy products for protein intake if not a cancer survivor.**

Substitutions/notes/symptoms
Indiscretions/distress/extra calories/etc.

____
____
____
____

Exercise	**Duration**

Total calories burned______

SMOKING IS DETRIMENTAL TO THE HEALTH OF MOST PEOPLE!

Thursday	**Breakfast**	**Lunch**	**Dinner**
	2 slices bacon	Shrimp Salad	4 ozs. pork
	1 blueberry muffin	Coleslaw	Peas
	1 cup kefir	Green Salad	Rice w/mushrooms
	Coffee/tea	Coffee/tea	Summer/Winter Squash

Snacks

8 ozs. carrot juice
1 cup strawberries
1 cup English walnuts
1 herbal tea

***Vegans replace dairy products with soy cheese and reconstituted non-dairy creamer. Every third day all weight managers should eat 1/2 cup beans, lentils, and other legumes.**

****Replace meat products with "chicken" (mushroom) tenders and meatballs (mushrooms). Full range of Quorn ® products is suggested for variety. You may also use soy products for protein intake if not a cancer survivor.**

Weigh-in Friday

Substitutions/notes/symptoms Indiscretions/distress/extra calories/etc. ____________________________ ____________________________ ____________________________ ____________________________ **Exercise Duration** **Total calories burned______**

DO I HAVE A BIOCHEMICAL THUMBPRINT? IS MINE DIFFERENT FROM ALL OTHERS? ***YES!!!!!!!!!!!***

Friday	**Breakfast**	**Lunch**	**Dinner**
	2 slices "lite" toast	**1 chef salad (chicken)**	**4 ozs. turkey**
	1 pat butter	**1 cup carrot juice**	**1 cup rice w/butter**
	½ cup pears	**1 cup blueberries**	**½ cup coleslaw**
	½ cup ricotta/c.cheese	**1 coffee/tea**	**8 ozs. cranberry juice**
	1 coffee/tea		

Snacks

2 kiwi fruits
1 cup pineapple juice
1 cup English walnuts
1 herbal tea

***Vegans replace dairy products with soy cheese and reconstituted non-dairy creamer. Every third day all weight managers should eat 1/2 cup beans, lentils, and other legumes.**

****Replace meat products with "chicken" (mushroom) tenders and meatballs (mushrooms). Full range of Quorn ® products is suggested for variety. You may also use soy products for protein intake if not a cancer survivor.**

Cycle 2 (4 days)

Substitutions/notes/symptoms Indiscretions/distress/extra calories/etc.

____

____

____

____

Exercise	**Duration**

Total calories burned______

COUNT WHAT YOU PUT IN YOUR MOUTH. YOU'LL BE GLAD YOU DID!

Saturday	**Breakast**	**Lunch**	**Dinner**
	1 ½ oz. cereal	4 ozs. chipped beef	4 ozs. fish
	* 4 ozs. milk	spinach salad	fiddlehead ferns
	1 cup blackberries	1 cup tangerine slices	Whole kernel corn
	1 English muffin	1 coffee/tea	Fresh parsnips
	1 coffee/tea		

Snacks

2 kiwi fruits
1 cup pineapple juice
1 cup English walnuts
1 herbal tea

*Vegans replace dairy products with soy cheese and reconstituted non-dairy creamer. Every third day all weight managers should eat 1/2 cup beans, lentils, and other legumes.

**Replace meat products with "chicken" (mushroom) tenders and meatballs (mushrooms). Full range of Quorn ® products is suggested for variety. You may also use soy products for protein intake if not a cancer survivor.

Substitutions/notes/symptoms
Indiscretions/distress/extra calories/etc.

____
____
____
____

Exercise Duration

Total calories burned______

HAVE I DONE MY BONES A FAVOR BY USING SOME FORM OF WEIGHT TRAINING EXERCISE?

Sunday	Breakfast	Lunch	Dinner
	2 eggs	Turkey sandwich	½ Cornish hen
	2 slices "lite" toast	Caesar salad	Macaroni & Cheese
	1 cup strawberries	½ cup salted s/flower seeds	Broccoli rabe
	6 ozs. orange juice	1 coffee/tea	Small green salad
	1 coffee/tea		8 ozs. elderberry juice

Snacks

1 oz. pita chips
Celery/Parsley/Apple Juice
5 tbsps. pumpkin seeds
Flavored water
1 herbal tea

***Vegans replace dairy products with soy cheese and reconstituted non-dairy creamer. Every third day all weight managers should eat 1/2 cup beans, lentils, and other legumes.**

****Replace meat products with "chicken" (mushroom) tenders and meatballs (mushrooms). Full range of Quorn ® products is suggested for variety. You may also use soy products for protein intake if not a cancer survivor.**

Substitutions/notes/symptoms Indiscretions/distress/extra calories/etc.
____
____
____
____
Exercise **Duration**
Total calories burned______

IF VITAMINS DON'T HELP ANYONE, TAKEN AS DIRECTED—ARE THEY LIKELY TO HARM ANYONE?

Monday	Breakast	Lunch	Dinner
	3 slices bacon	Grilled Jumbo Shrimp	4 ozs. pork roast
	1 raspberry muffin	Medium Salad w/dressing	Yams
	1 cup raspberries	½ cup salted s/flower seeds	Cauliflower
	6 ozs. pineapple j.	1 coffee/tea	Small green salad
	1 coffee/tea		8 ozs. apricot nectar

Snacks

4 tbsps. peanuts
½ cup peaches
1 vanilla yogurt
1 herbal tea

*Vegans replace dairy products with soy cheese and reconstituted non-dairy creamer. Every third day all weight managers should eat 1/2 cup beans, lentils, and other legumes.

**Replace meat products with "chicken" (mushroom) tenders and meatballs (mushrooms). Full range of Quorn ® products is suggested for variety. You may also use soy products for protein intake if not a cancer survivor.

Weigh-In: Tuesday

Cycle 3 (4 days)

Substitutions/notes/symptoms Indiscretions/distress/extra calories/etc.
____
____
____
____
Exercise Duration
Total calories burned______

ARE THERE ANY MIRACLES LEFT? EXERCISE IS A MIRACLE!

Tuesday	Breakfast	Lunch	Dinner
	1 ½ ounce cereal	**6 ozs. Tuna salad w/ toast	**4 ozs. Beef
	*4 ozs. milk	Spinach Salad	Asparagus
	1 cup canned peaches	Fruit cocktail	Rice pasta
	1 English muffin	Elderberry juice	Parsnips
	W/all fruit spread	Coffee/tea	
	Coffee/tea		

Snacks

Veggie chips (1 oz.)
8 ozs. kefir
4 tbsps. peanuts
1 herbal tea

***Vegans replace dairy products with soy cheese and reconstituted non-dairy creamer. Every third day all weight managers should eat 1/2 cup beans, lentils, and other legumes.**

**** Vegans/Vegetarians replace meat products with "chicken" (mushroom) tenders and meatballs (mushrooms). Full range of Quorn ® products is suggested for variety. You may also use soy products for protein intake if not a cancer survivor.**

Substitutions/notes/symptoms Indiscretions/distress/extra calories/etc. ____________________ ____________________ ____________________ ____________________ **Exercise Duration** **Total calories burned______**

EXCESSIVE DRINKING IS DETRIMENTAL TO THE HEALTH OF MOST PEOPLE!

Wednesday	Breakfast	Lunch	Dinner
	egg beaters® omelet scrambled with peppers/ onions /sour cream dollop	Turkey Salad	4-6 ozs. fish
		Green salad	Zucchini
		½ cup pineapple	Carrots
	1 slice toast w/butter	Coffee/tea	½ cup buttered pasta
	Coffee/tea	Raw carrot juice	

Snacks

1 oz. potato chips
8 elderberry juice
½ cup canned/fresh apricots
1 herbal tea

***Vegans replace dairy products with soy cheese and non-dairy creamer reconstituted.**

****Replace meat products with "chicken" (mushroom) tenders and meatballs (mushrooms). Full range of Quorn ® products is suggested for variety. You may also use soy products for protein intake if not a cancer survivor.**

Substitutions/notes/symptoms
Indiscretions/distress/extra calories/etc.

____
____
____
____

Exercise	**Duration**

Total calories burned______

IF YOU THINK THE FOOD CHAIN IS AS HEALTHY TODAY AS IT WAS A DECADE OR SO AGO, ASK THE NUCLEAR SCIENTISTS AND FARMERS OF TODAY!

Thursday	**Breakfast**	**Lunch**	**Dinner**
	2 slices bacon	Shrimp Salad	4 ozs. pork
	1 blueberry muffin	Coleslaw	Peas
	1 cup kefir	Green Salad	Rice w/mushrooms
	Coffee/tea	Coffee/tea	Summer/Winter Squash

Snacks

8 ozs. carrot juice
1 cup strawberries
1 cup English walnuts
1 herbal tea

***Vegans replace dairy products with soy cheese and reconstituted non-dairy creamer. Every third day all weight managers should eat 1/2 cup beans, lentils, and other legumes.**

****Replace meat products with "chicken" (mushroom) tenders and meatballs (mushrooms). Full range of Quorn ® products is suggested for variety. You may also use soy products for protein intake if not a cancer survivor.**

Substitutions/notes/symptoms Indiscretions/distress/extra calories/etc.

____
____
____
____

Exercise Duration

Total calories burned______

IS IT BETTER BECAUSE IT IS FRESH? YES, IF IT IS PROPERLY CLEANED!

Friday	Breakfast	Lunch	Dinner
	2 slices "lite" toast	1 chef salad (chicken)	4 ozs. turkey
	1 pat butter	1 cup carrot juice	1 cup rice w/butter
	½ cup pears	1 cup blueberries	½ cup coleslaw
	½ cup ricotta/c.cheese	1 coffee/tea	8 ozs. cranberry juice
	1 coffee/tea		

Snacks

2 kiwi fruits
1 cup pineapple juice
1 cup English walnuts
1 herbal tea

***Vegans replace dairy products with soy cheese and reconstituted non-dairy creamer. Every third day all weight managers should eat 1/2 cup beans, lentils, and other legumes.**

****Replace meat products with "chicken" (mushroom) tenders and meatballs (mushrooms). Full range of Quorn ® products is suggested for variety. You may also use soy products for protein intake if not a cancer survivor.**

Weigh-in: Saturday

Cycle 4 (4 days)

Substitutions/notes/symptoms
Indiscretions/distress/extra calories/etc.

____
____
____
____

Exercise Duration

Total calories burned______

HAVE I DONE MY EXERCISE TODAY?

Saturday	Breakast	Lunch	Dinner
	1 ½ oz. cereal	4 ozs. chipped beef	4 ozs. fish
	* 4 ozs. milk	spinach salad	fiddlehead ferns
	1 cup blackberries	1 cup tangerine slices	Whole kernel corn
	1 English muffin	1 coffee/tea	Fresh parsnips
	1 coffee/tea		

Snacks

½ cup lentils
2 kiwi fruits
1 cup pineapple juice
1 cup English walnuts
1 herbal tea

***Vegans replace dairy products with soy cheese and reconstituted non-dairy creamer. Every third day all weight managers should eat 1/2 cup beans, lentils, and other legumes.**

****Replace meat products with "chicken" (mushroom) tenders and meatballs (mushrooms). Full range of Quorn ® products is suggested for variety. You may also use soy products for protein intake if not a cancer survivor.**

Substitutions/notes/symptoms
Indiscretions/distress/extra calories/etc.

____

____

____

____

Exercise **Duration**

Total calories burned______

HAVE I DONE MY BONES A FAVOR BY USING SOME FORM OF WEIGHT TRAINING EXERCISE?

Sunday	Breakfast	Lunch	Dinner
	2 eggs	Turkey sandwich	½ Cornish hen
	1 slice "lite" toast	Caesar salad	Macaroni & Cheese
	1 cup strawberries	½ cup salted s/flower seeds	Broccoli rabe
	6 ozs. orange juice	1 coffee/tea	Small green salad
	1 coffee/tea		8 ozs. elderberry j.

Snacks

1 oz. pita chips
Celery/Parsley/Apple Juice
5 tbsps. pumpkin seeds
Flavored water
1 herbal tea

***Vegans replace dairy products with soy cheese and reconstituted non-dairy creamer. Every third day all weight managers should eat 1/2 cup beans, lentils, and other legumes.**

****Replace meat products with "chicken" (mushroom) tenders and meatballs (mushrooms). Full range of Quorn ® products is suggested for variety. You may also use soy products for protein intake if not a cancer survivor.**

Substitutions/notes/symptoms
Indiscretions/distress/extra calories/etc.

____
____
____
____

Exercise **Duration**

Total calories burned______

EXCESSIVE DRINKING IS DETRIMENTAL TO THE HEALTH OF MOST PEOPLE!

Monday	Breakast	Lunch	Dinner
	3 slices bacon	Grilled Jumbo Shrimp	4 ozs. pork roast
	1 raspberry muffin	Medium Salad w/dressing	Yams
	1 cup raspberries	½ cup salted s/flower seeds	Cauliflower
	6 ozs. pineapple j.	1 coffee/tea	Small green salad
	1 coffee/tea		8 ozs. apricot nectar

Snacks

4 tbsps. peanuts
½ cup peaches
1 vanilla yogurt
1 herbal tea

***Vegans replace dairy products with soy cheese and reconstituted non-dairy creamer. Every third day all weight managers should eat 1/2 cup beans, lentils, and other legumes.**

****Replace meat products with "chicken" (mushroom) tenders and meatballs (mushrooms). Full range of Quorn ® products is suggested for variety. You may also use soy products for protein intake if not a cancer survivor.**

Weigh in: Wednesday

Substitutions/notes/symptoms Indiscretions/distress/extra calories/etc. ____________________________ ____________________________ ____________________________ **Exercise Duration** **Total calories burned______**

EXCESSIVE DRINKING IS DETRIMENTAL TO THE HEALTH OF MOST PEOPLE!

Tuesday	Breakfast	Lunch	Dinner
	1 ½ ounce cereal	**6 ozs. Tuna salad w/ toast	**4 ozs. Beef
	*4 ozs. milk	Spinach Salad	Asparagus
	1 cup canned peaches	Fruit cocktail	Rice pasta
	1 English muffin W/all fruit spread	Elderberry juice	Parsnips
	Coffee/tea	Coffee/tea	

Snacks

1 oz. veggie chips
½ cup black beans
8 ozs. kefir
4 tbsps. peanuts
1 herbal tea

*Vegans replace dairy products with soy cheese and reconstituted non-dairy creamer. Every third day all weight managers should eat 1/2 cup beans, lentils, and other legumes.

** Vegans/Vegetarians replace meat products with "chicken" (mushroom) tenders and meatballs (mushrooms). Full range of Quorn ® products is suggested for variety. You may also use soy products for protein intake if not a cancer survivor.

Cycle 5 (4 days)

Substitutions/notes/symptoms Indiscretions/distress/extra calories/etc.

____

____

____

____

Exercise Duration

Total calories burned______

DO I REALLY NEED VITAMINS IS LIKE ASKING DO I REALLY NEED INSURANCE!

Wednesday	Breakfast	Lunch	Dinner
	egg beaters® omelet scrambled with peppers/ onions /sour cream dollop	Turkey Salad	4-6 ozs. fish
	1 slice toast w/butter	Green salad	Zucchini
	Coffee/tea	½ cup pineapple	Carrots
		Coffee/tea	½ cup buttered pasta
		Raw carrot juice	

Snacks

1 oz. potato chips
8 elderberry juice
½ cup canned/fresh apricots
1 herbal tea

***Vegans replace dairy products with soy cheese and non-dairy creamer reconstituted.**

****Replace meat products with "chicken" (mushroom) tenders and meatballs (mushrooms). Full range of Quorn ® products is suggested for variety. You may also use soy products for protein intake if not a cancer survivor.**

Substitutions/notes/symptoms Indiscretions/distress/extra calories/etc.

____

____

____

____

Exercise	**Duration**

Total calories burned______

IF YOU THINK THE FOOD CHAIN IS AS HEALTHY TODAY AS IT WAS A DECADE OR SO AGO, ASK THE NUCLEAR SCIENTISTS AND FARMERS OF TODAY!

Thursday	**Breakfast**	**Lunch**	**Dinner**
	2 slices bacon	**Shrimp Salad**	**4 ozs. pork**
	1 blueberry muffin	**Coleslaw**	**Peas**
	1 cup kefir	**Green Salad**	**Rice w/mushrooms**
	Coffee/tea	**Coffee/tea**	**Summer/Winter Squash**

Snacks

8 ozs. carrot juice
1 cup strawberries
1 cup English walnuts
1 herbal tea

***Vegans replace dairy products with soy cheese and reconstituted non-dairy creamer. Every third day all weight managers should eat 1/2 cup beans, lentils, and other legumes.**

****Replace meat products with "chicken" (mushroom) tenders and meatballs (mushrooms). Full range of Quorn ® products is suggested for variety. You may also use soy products for protein intake if not a cancer survivor.**

Substitutions/notes/symptoms Indiscretions/distress/extra calories/etc.
____
____
____
____
Exercise **Duration**
Total calories burned______

IS IT BETTER BECAUSE IT IS FRESH? YES, IF IT IS PROPERLY CLEANED!

Friday	Breakfast	Lunch	Dinner
	2 slices"lite" toast 1 pat butter ½ cup pears ½ cup ricotta/c.cheese 1 coffee/tea	1 chef salad (chicken) 1 cup carrot juice 1 cup blueberries 1 coffee/tea	4 ozs. turkey 1 cup rice w/butter ½ cup coleslaw 8 ozs. cranberry juice

Snacks

2 kiwi fruits
1 cup pineapple juice
1 cup English walnuts
1 herbal tea

***Vegans replace dairy products with soy cheese and reconstituted non-dairy creamer. Every third day all weight managers should eat 1/2 cup beans, lentils, and other legumes.**

****Replace meat products with "chicken" (mushroom) tenders and meatballs (mushrooms). Full range of Quorn ® products is suggested for variety. You may also use soy products for protein intake if not a cancer survivor.**

Substitutions/notes/symptoms Indiscretions/distress/extra calories/etc.
____
____
____
____
Exercise **Duration**
Total calories burned______

HAVE I DONE MY EXERCISE TODAY?

Saturday	Breakast	Lunch	Dinner
	1 ½ oz. cereal	4 ozs. chipped beef	4 ozs. fish
	* 4 ozs. milk	spinach salad	fiddlehead ferns
	1 cup blackberries	1 cup tangerine slices	Whole kernel corn
	1 English muffin	1 coffee/tea	Fresh parsnips
	1 coffee/tea		

Snacks

2 kiwi fruits
1 cup pineapple juice
1 cup English walnuts
1 herbal tea

***Vegans replace dairy products with soy cheese and reconstituted non-dairy creamer. Every third day all weight managers should eat 1/2 cup beans, lentils, and other legumes.**

****Replace meat products with "chicken" (mushroom) tenders and meatballs (mushrooms). Full range of Quorn ® products is suggested for variety. You may also use soy products for protein intake if not a cancer survivor.**

Weigh In: Sunday

Cycle 7 (4 days)

Substitutions/notes/symptoms Indiscretions/distress/extra calories/etc.

____
____
____
____

Exercise	**Duration**

Total calories burned______

HAVE I DONE MY BONES A FAVOR BY USING SOME FORM OF WEIGHT TRAINING EXERCISE?

Sunday	Breakfast	Lunch	Dinner
	2 eggs	Turkey sandwich	½ Cornish hen
	1 slice "lite" toast	Caesar salad	Macaroni & Cheese
	1 cup strawberries	½ cup salted s/flower seeds	Broccoli rabe
	6 ozs. orange juice	1 coffee/tea	Small green salad
	1 coffee/tea		8 ozs. elderberry j.

Snacks

1 oz. pita chips
½ cup pinto beans
Celery/Parsley/Apple Juice

***Vegans replace dairy products with soy cheese and reconstituted non-dairy creamer. Every third day all weight managers should eat 1/2 cup beans, lentils, and other legumes.**

****Replace meat products with "chicken" (mushroom) tenders and meatballs (mushrooms). Full range of Quorn ® products is suggested for variety. You may also use soy products for protein intake if not a cancer survivor.**

Substitutions/notes/symptoms
Indiscretions/distress/extra calories/etc.

____
____
____
____

Exercise **Duration**

Total calories burned______

EXCESSIVE DRINKING IS DETRIMENTAL TO THE HEALTH OF MOST PEOPLE!

Monday	Breakast	Lunch	Dinner
	3 slices bacon	Grilled Jumbo Shrimp	4 ozs. pork roast
	1 raspberry muffin	Medium Salad w/dressing	Yams
	1 cup raspberries	½ cup salted s/flower seeds	Cauliflower
	6 ozs. pineapple j.	1 coffee/tea	Small green salad
	1 coffee/tea		8 ozs. apricot nectar

Snacks

4 tbsps. peanuts
½ cup peaches
1 vanilla yogurt
1 herbal tea

***Vegans replace dairy products with soy cheese and reconstituted non-dairy creamer. Every third day all weight managers should eat 1/2 cup beans, lentils, and other legumes.**

****Replace meat products with "chicken" (mushroom) tenders and meatballs (mushrooms). Full range of Quorn ® products is suggested for variety. You may also use soy products for protein intake if not a cancer survivor.**

Substitutions/notes/symptoms Indiscretions/distress/extra calories/etc.
____
____
____
____
Exercise **Duration**
Total calories burned______

EXCESSIVE DRINKING IS DETRIMENTAL TO THE HEALTH OF MOST PEOPLE!

Tuesday	Breakfast	Lunch	Dinner
	1 ½ ounce cereal	**6 ozs. Tuna salad w/ toast	**4 ozs. Beef
	*4 ozs. milk	Spinach Salad	Asparagus
	1 cup canned peaches	Fruit cocktail	Rice pasta
	1 English muffin	Elderberry juice	Parsnips
	W/all fruit spread	Coffee/tea	
	Coffee/tea		

Snacks

Veggie chips
8 ozs. kefir
4 tbsps. peanuts
1 herbal tea

*Vegans replace dairy products with soy cheese and reconstituted non-dairy creamer. Every third day all weight managers should eat 1/2 cup beans, lentils, and other legumes.

** Vegans/Vegetarians replace meat products with "chicken" (mushroom) tenders and meatballs (mushrooms). Full range of Quorn ® products is suggested for variety. You may also use soy products for protein intake if not a cancer survivor.

Substitutions/notes/symptoms Indiscretions/distress/extra calories/etc. __________________________ __________________________ __________________________ __________________________ **Exercise Duration** **Total calories burned______**

DO I REALLY NEED VITAMINS IS LIKE ASKING DO I REALLY NEED INSURANCE!

Wednesday	Breakfast	Lunch	Dinner
	egg beaters® omelet scrambled with peppers/ onions /sour cream dollop	Turkey Salad	4-6 ozs. fish
		Green salad	Zucchini
		½ cup pineapple	Carrots
	1 slice toast w/butter	Coffee/tea	½ cup buttered pasta
	Coffee/tea	Raw carrot juice	

Snacks

1 oz. potato chips
8 ozs. elderberry juice
½ cup canned/fresh apricots
1 herbal tea

***Vegans replace dairy products with soy cheese and non-dairy creamer reconstituted.**

****Replace meat products with "chicken" (mushroom) tenders and meatballs (mushrooms). Full range of Quorn ® products is suggested for variety. You may also use soy products for protein intake if not a cancer survivor.**

Weigh-in: Thursday

Cycle 8 (4 Days)

Substitutions/notes/symptoms Indiscretions/distress/extra calories/etc.
____
____
____
____
Exercise **Duration**
Total calories burned______

IF YOU THINK THE FOOD CHAIN IS AS HEALTHY TODAY AS IT WAS A DECADE OR SO AGO, ASK THE NUCLEAR SCIENTISTS AND FARMERS OF TODAY!

Thursday	Breakfast	Lunch	Dinner
	2 slices bacon	Shrimp Salad	4 ozs. pork
	1 blueberry muffin	Coleslaw	Peas
	1 cup kefir	Green Salad	Rice w/mushrooms
	Coffee/tea	Coffee/tea	Summer/Winter Squash

Snacks

½ cup beans (any variety)
8 ozs. carrot juice
1 cup strawberries
1 cup English walnuts
1 herbal tea

***Vegans replace dairy products with soy cheese and reconstituted non-dairy creamer. Every third day all weight managers should eat 1/2 cup beans, lentils, and other legumes.**

****Replace meat products with "chicken" (mushroom) tenders and meatballs (mushrooms). Full range of Quorn ® products is suggested for variety. You may also use soy products for protein intake if not a cancer survivor.**

Substitutions/notes/symptoms Indiscretions/distress/extra calories/etc.
____
____
____
____
Exercise Duration
Total calories burned______

IS IT BETTER BECAUSE IT IS FRESH? YES, IF IT IS PROPERLY CLEANED!

Friday	Breakfast	Lunch	Dinner
	2 slices "lite" toast 1 pat butter ½ cup pears ½ cup ricotta/c.cheese 1 coffee/tea	1 chef salad (chicken) 1 cup carrot juice 1 cup blueberries 1 coffee/tea	4 ozs. turkey 1 cup rice w/butter ½ cup coleslaw 8 ozs. cranberry juice

Snacks

2 kiwi fruits
1 cup pineapple juice
1 cup English walnuts
1 herbal tea

*Vegans replace dairy products with soy cheese and reconstituted non-dairy creamer. Every third day all weight managers should eat 1/2 cup beans, lentils, and other legumes.

**Replace meat products with "chicken" (mushroom) tenders and meatballs (mushrooms). Full range of Quorn ® products is suggested for variety. You may also use soy products for protein intake if not a cancer survivor.

Substitutions/notes/symptoms
Indiscretions/distress/extra calories/etc.

____
____
____
____

Exercise Duration

Total calories burned______

COUNT WHAT YOU PUT IN YOUR MOUTH. YOU'LL BE GLAD YOU DID!

Saturday	Breakast	Lunch	Dinner
	1 ½ oz. cereal	4 ozs. chipped beef	4 ozs. fish
	* 4 ozs. milk	spinach salad	fiddlehead ferns
	1 cup blackberries	1 cup tangerine slices	Whole kernel corn
	1 English muffin	1 coffee/tea	Fresh parsnips
	1 coffee/tea		

Snacks

2 kiwi fruits
1 cup pineapple juice
1 cup English walnuts
1 herbal tea

***Vegans replace dairy products with soy cheese and reconstituted non-dairy creamer. Every third day all weight managers should eat 1/2 cup beans, lentils, and other legumes.**

****Replace meat products with "chicken" (mushroom) tenders and meatballs (mushrooms). Full range of Quorn ® products is suggested for variety. You may also use soy products for protein intake if not a cancer survivor.**

Substitutions/notes/symptoms
Indiscretions/distress/extra calories/etc.

____
____
____
____

Exercise Duration

Total calories burned______

EXCESSIVE DRINKING IS DETRIMENTAL TO THE HEALTH OF MOST PEOPLE!

Sunday	Breakfast	Lunch	Dinner
	2 eggs	Turkey sandwich	½ Cornish hen
	1 slice "lite" toast	Caesar salad	Macaroni & Cheese
	1 cup strawberries	½ cup salted s/flower seeds	Broccoli rabe
	6 ozs. orange juice	1 coffee/tea	Small green salad
	1 coffee/tea		8 ozs. elderberry j.

Snacks

1 oz. pita chips
Celery/Parsley/Apple Juice
5 tbsps. pumpkin seeds
Flavored water
1 herbal tea

***Vegans replace dairy products with soy cheese and reconstituted non-dairy creamer. Every third day all weight managers should eat 1/2 cup beans, lentils, and other legumes.**

****Replace meat products with "chicken" (mushroom) tenders and meatballs (mushrooms). Full range of Quorn ® products is suggested for variety. You may also use soy products for protein intake if not a cancer survivor.**

Weigh-in: Monday

Cycle 9 (4 days)

Substitutions/notes/symptoms Indiscretions/distress/extra calories/etc.
____
____
____
____
Exercise Duration
Total calories burned______

EXCESSIVE DRINKING IS DETRIMENTAL TO THE HEALTH OF MOST PEOPLE!

Monday	Breakast	Lunch	Dinner
	3 slices bacon	Grilled Jumbo Shrimp	4 ozs. pork roast
	1 raspberry muffin	Medium Salad w/dressing	Yams
	1 cup raspberries	½ cup salted s/flower seeds	Cauliflower
	6 ozs. pineapple j.	1 coffee/tea	Small green salad
	1 coffee/tea		8 ozs. apricot nectar

Snacks

½ cup beans (any variety)
½ cup peaches
1 vanilla yogurt
1 herbal tea

***Vegans replace dairy products with soy cheese and reconstituted non-dairy creamer. Every third day all weight managers should eat 1/2 cup beans, lentils, and other legumes.**

****Replace meat products with "chicken" (mushroom) tenders and meatballs (mushrooms). Full range of Quorn ® products is suggested for variety. You may also use soy products for protein intake if not a cancer survivor.**

Substitutions/notes/symptoms
Indiscretions/distress/extra calories/etc.

____
____
____
____

Exercise	**Duration**

Total calories burned______

EXCESSIVE DRINKING IS DETRIMENTAL TO THE HEALTH OF MOST PEOPLE!

Tuesday	**Breakfast**	**Lunch**	**Dinner**
	1 ½ ounce cereal	****6 ozs. Tuna salad w/ toast**	****4 ozs. Beef**
	***4 ozs. milk**	**Spinach Salad**	**Asparagus**
	1 cup canned peaches	**Fruit cocktail**	**Rice pasta**
	1 English muffin	**Elderberry juice**	**Parsnips**
	W/all fruit spread	**Coffee/tea**	
	Coffee/tea		

Snacks

1 oz. veggie chips
8 ozs. kefir
4 tbsps. peanuts
1 herbal tea

***Vegans replace dairy products with soy cheese and reconstituted non-dairy creamer. Every third day all weight managers should eat 1/2 cup beans, lentils, and other legumes.**

**** Vegans/Vegetarians replace meat products with "chicken" (mushroom) tenders and meatballs (mushrooms). Full range of Quorn ® products is suggested for variety. You may also use soy products for protein intake if not a cancer survivor.**

Substitutions/notes/symptoms Indiscretions/distress/extra calories/etc.

____

____

____

____

Exercise	**Duration**

Total calories burned______

DO I REALLY NEED VITAMINS IS LIKE ASKING DO I REALLY NEED INSURANCE!

Wednesday	**Breakfast**	**Lunch**	**Dinner**
	egg beaters® omelet scrambled with peppers/ onions /sour cream dollop	Turkey Salad	4-6 ozs. fish
		Green salad	Zucchini
		½ cup pineapple	Carrots
	1 slice toast w/butter	Coffee/tea	½ cup buttered pasta
	Coffee/tea	Raw carrot juice	

Snacks

1 oz. potato chips
8 elderberry juice
½ cup canned/fresh apricots
1 herbal tea

***Vegans replace dairy products with soy cheese and non-dairy creamer reconstituted.**

****Replace meat products with "chicken" (mushroom) tenders and meatballs (mushrooms). Full range of Quorn ® products is suggested for variety. You may also use soy products for protein intake if not a cancer survivor.**

Substitutions/notes/symptoms Indiscretions/distress/extra calories/etc.

____

____

____

____

Exercise Duration

Total calories burned______

IF YOU THINK THE FOOD CHAIN IS AS HEALTHY TODAY AS IT WAS A DECADE OR SO AGO, ASK THE NUCLEAR SCIENTISTS AND FARMERS OF TODAY!

Thursday	Breakfast	Lunch	Dinner
	2 slices bacon	Shrimp Salad	4 ozs. pork
	1 blueberry muffin	Coleslaw	Peas
	1 cup kefir	Green Salad	Rice w/mushrooms
	Coffee/tea	Coffee/tea	Summer/Winter Squash

Snacks

8 ozs. carrot juice
1 cup strawberries
1 cup English walnuts
1 herbal tea

***Vegans replace dairy products with soy cheese and reconstituted non-dairy creamer. Every third day all weight managers should eat 1/2 cup beans, lentils, and other legumes.**

****Replace meat products with "chicken" (mushroom) tenders and meatballs (mushrooms). Full range of Quorn ® products is suggested for variety. You may also use soy products for protein intake if not a cancer survivor.**

Weigh-in: Friday

Cycle 10 (4 days)

Substitutions/notes/symptoms Indiscretions/distress/extra calories/etc.

____
____
____
____

Exercise Duration

Total calories burned______

IS IT BETTER BECAUSE IT IS FRESH? YES, IF IT IS PROPERLY CLEANED!

Friday	Breakfast	Lunch	Dinner
	2 slices "lite" toast 1 pat butter ½ cup pears ½ cup ricotta/c.cheese 1 coffee/tea	1 chef salad (chicken) 1 cup carrot juice 1 cup blueberries 1 coffee/tea	4 ozs. turkey 1 cup rice w/butter ½ cup coleslaw 8 ozs. cranberry juice

Snacks

2 kiwi fruits
1 cup lentils
1 cup pineapple juice
1 cup English walnuts
1 herbal tea

*Vegans replace dairy products with soy cheese and reconstituted non-dairy creamer. Every third day all weight managers should eat 1/2 cup beans, lentils, and other legumes.

**Replace meat products with "chicken" (mushroom) tenders and meatballs (mushrooms). Full range of Quorn ® products is suggested for variety. You may also use soy products for protein intake if not a cancer survivor.

Substitutions/notes/symptoms
Indiscretions/distress/extra calories/etc.

____
____
____
____

Exercise Duration

Total calories burned______

HAVE I DONE MY EXERCISE TODAY?

Saturday	Breakast	Lunch	Dinner
	1 ½ oz. cereal	4 ozs. chipped beef	4 ozs. fish
	* 4 ozs. milk	spinach salad	fiddlehead ferns
	1 cup blackberries	1 cup tangerine slices	Whole kernel corn
	1 English muffin	1 coffee/tea	Fresh parsnips
	1 coffee/tea		

Snacks

2 kiwi fruits
1 cup pineapple juice
1 cup English walnuts
1 herbal tea

***Vegans replace dairy products with soy cheese and reconstituted non-dairy creamer. Every third day all weight managers should eat 1/2 cup beans, lentils, and other legumes.**

****Replace meat products with "chicken" (mushroom) tenders and meatballs (mushrooms). Full range of Quorn ® products is suggested for variety. You may also use soy products for protein intake if not a cancer survivor.**

Substitutions/notes/symptoms Indiscretions/distress/extra calories/etc.

____

____

____

____

Exercise	**Duration**

Total calories burned______

HAVE I DONE MY BONES A FAVOR BY USING SOME FORM OF WEIGHT TRAINING EXERCISE?

Sunday	**Breakfast**	**Lunch**	**Dinner**
	2 eggs	Turkey sandwich	½ Cornish hen
	1 slice "lite" toast	Caesar salad	Macaroni & Cheese
	1 cup strawberries	½ cup salted s/flower seeds	Broccoli rabe
	6 ozs. orange juice	1 coffee/tea	Small green salad
	1 coffee/tea		8 ozs. elderberry juice

Snacks

1 oz. pita chips
Celery/Parsley/Apple Juice
5 tbsps. pumpkin seeds
Flavored water
1 herbal tea

***Vegans replace dairy products with soy cheese and reconstituted non-dairy creamer. Every third day all weight managers should eat 1/2 cup beans, lentils, and other legumes.**

****Replace meat products with "chicken" (mushroom) tenders and meatballs (mushrooms). Full range of Quorn ® products is suggested for variety. You may also use soy products for protein intake if not a cancer survivor.**

Substitutions/notes/symptoms Indiscretions/distress/extra calories/etc.
____
____
____
____
Exercise **Duration**
Total calories burned______

EXCESSIVE DRINKING IS DETRIMENTAL TO THE HEALTH OF MOST PEOPLE!

Monday	Breakast	Lunch	Dinner
	3 slices bacon	Grilled Jumbo Shrimp	4 ozs. pork roast
	1 raspberry muffin	Medium Salad w/dressing	Yams
	1 cup raspberries	½ cup salted s/flower seeds	Cauliflower
	6 ozs. pineapple j.	1 coffee/tea	Small green salad
	1 coffee/tea		8 ozs. apricot nectar

Snacks

4 tbsps. macadamia nuts
½ cup peaches
1 vanilla yogurt
1 herbal tea

*Vegans replace dairy products with soy cheese and reconstituted non-dairy creamer. Every third day all weight managers should eat 1/2 cup beans, lentils, and other legumes.

**Replace meat products with "chicken" (mushroom) tenders and meatballs (mushrooms). Full range of Quorn ® products is suggested for variety. You may also use soy products for protein intake if not a cancer survivor.

Weigh-in: Tuesday

Cycle 11 (4 days)

Substitutions/notes/symptoms Indiscretions/distress/extra calories/etc.
____
____
____
____
Exercise **Duration**
Total calories burned______

DID I LIKE WHAT I ATE? IS IT SURE TO SATISFY MY PERSONAL CRAVINGS? WAS IT HEALTHY?

Tuesday	Breakfast	Lunch	Dinner
	1 ½ ounce cereal *4 ozs. milk 1 cup canned peaches 1 English muffin W/all fruit spread Coffee/tea	**6 ozs. Tuna salad/toast Spinach Salad Fruit cocktail Elderberry juice Coffee/tea	**4 ozs. Beef Asparagus Rice pasta Parsnips

Snacks

½ cup lentils
1 oz. veggie chips
8 ozs. kefir
4 tbsps. peanuts
1 herbal tea

*Vegans replace dairy products with soy cheese and reconstituted non-dairy creamer. Every third day all weight managers should eat 1/2 cup beans, lentils, and other legumes.

** Vegans/Vegetarians replace meat products with "chicken" (mushroom) tenders and meatballs (mushrooms). Full range of Quorn ® products is suggested for variety. You may also use soy products for protein intake if not a cancer survivor.

Substitutions/notes/symptoms
Indiscretions/distress/extra calories/etc.

____

____

____

____

Exercise Duration

Total calories burned______

DO I REALLY NEED VITAMINS IS LIKE ASKING DO I REALLY NEED INSURANCE!

Wednesday	Breakfast	Lunch	Dinner
	egg beaters® omelet scrambled with peppers/ onions /sour cream dollop	Turkey Salad	4-6 ozs. fish
	1 slice toast w/butter	Green salad	Zucchini
	Coffee/tea	½ cup pineapple	Carrots
		Coffee/tea	½ cup buttered pasta
		Raw carrot juice	

Snacks

1 oz. potato chips
8 elderberry juice
½ cup canned/fresh apricots
1 herbal tea

***Vegans replace dairy products with soy cheese and non-dairy creamer reconstituted.**

****Replace meat products with "chicken" (mushroom) tenders and meatballs (mushrooms). Full range of Quorn ® products is suggested for variety. You may also use soy products for protein intake if not a cancer survivor.**

Substitutions/notes/symptoms Indiscretions/distress/extra calories/etc.
____
____
____
____
Exercise Duration
Total calories burned______

IF YOU THINK THE FOOD CHAIN IS AS HEALTHY TODAY AS IT WAS A DECADE OR SO AGO, ASK THE NUCLEAR SCIENTISTS AND FARMERS OF TODAY!

Thursday	Breakfast	Lunch	Dinner
	2 slices bacon	Shrimp Salad	4 ozs. pork
	1 blueberry muffin	Coleslaw	Peas
	1 cup kefir	Green Salad	Rice w/mushrooms
	Coffee/tea	Coffee/tea	Summer/Winter Squash

Snacks

8 ozs. carrot juice
1 cup strawberries
1 cup English walnuts
1 herbal tea

***Vegans replace dairy products with soy cheese and reconstituted non-dairy creamer. Every third day all weight managers should eat 1/2 cup beans, lentils, and other legumes.**

****Replace meat products with "chicken" (mushroom) tenders and meatballs (mushrooms). Full range of Quorn ® products is suggested for variety. You may also use soy products for protein intake if not a cancer survivor.**

Substitutions/notes/symptoms Indiscretions/distress/extra calories/etc.
____
____
____
____
Exercise Duration
Total calories burned______

IS IT BETTER BECAUSE IT IS FRESH? YES, IF IT IS PROPERLY CLEANED!

Friday	Breakfast	Lunch	Dinner
	2 slices "lite" toast	1 chef salad (chicken)	4 ozs. turkey
	1 pat butter	1 cup carrot juice	1 cup rice w/butter
	½ cup pears	1 cup blueberries	½ cup coleslaw
	½ cup ricotta/c.cheese	1 coffee/tea	8 ozs. cranberry juice
	1 coffee/tea		

Snacks

2 kiwi fruits
1 cup pineapple juice
1 cup English walnuts
1 herbal tea

*Vegans replace dairy products with soy cheese and reconstituted non-dairy creamer. Every third day all weight managers should eat 1/2 cup beans, lentils, and other legumes.

**Replace meat products with "chicken" (mushroom) tenders and meatballs (mushrooms). Full range of Quorn ® products is suggested for variety. You may also use soy products for protein intake if not a cancer survivor.

Weigh-in: Saturday

Cycle 12 (4 days)

Substitutions/notes/symptoms
Indiscretions/distress/extra calories/etc.

____
____
____
____

Exercise	**Duration**

Total calories burned______

HAVE I DONE MY EXERCISE TODAY?

Saturday	**Breakast**	**Lunch**	**Dinner**
	1 ½ oz. cereal	4 ozs. chipped beef	4 ozs. fish
	* 4 ozs. milk	spinach salad	fiddlehead ferns
	1 cup blackberries	1 cup tangerine slices	Whole kernel corn
	1 English muffin	1 coffee/tea	Fresh parsnips
	1 coffee/tea		

Snacks

2 kiwi fruits
½ cup beasn
1 cup pineapple juice
1 cup English walnuts
1 herbal tea

***Vegans replace dairy products with soy cheese and reconstituted non-dairy creamer. Every third day all weight managers should eat 1/2 cup beans, lentils, and other legumes.**

****Replace meat products with "chicken" (mushroom) tenders and meatballs (mushrooms). Full range of Quorn ® products is suggested for variety. You may also use soy products for protein intake if not a cancer survivor.**

Substitutions/notes/symptoms Indiscretions/distress/extra calories/etc.

____
____
____
____

Exercise	**Duration**

Total calories burned______

HAVE I DONE MY BONES A FAVOR BY USING SOME FORM OF WEIGHT TRAINING EXERCISE?

Sunday	**Breakfast**	**Lunch**	**Dinner**
	2 eggs	Turkey sandwich	½ Cornish hen
	1 slice "lite" toast	Caesar salad	Macaroni & Cheese
	1 cup strawberries	½ cup salted s/flower seeds	Broccoli rabe
	6 ozs. orange juice	1 coffee/tea	Small green salad
	1 coffee/tea		8 ozs. elderberry juice

Snacks

1 oz. pita chips
Celery/Parsley/Apple Juice
5 tbsps. pumpkin seeds
Flavored water
1 herbal tea

***Vegans replace dairy products with soy cheese and reconstituted non-dairy creamer. Every third day all weight managers should eat 1/2 cup beans, lentils, and other legumes.**

****Replace meat products with "chicken" (mushroom) tenders and meatballs (mushrooms). Full range of Quorn ® products is suggested for variety. You may also use soy products for protein intake if not a cancer survivor.**

Substitutions/notes/symptoms
Indiscretions/distress/extra calories/etc.

____
____
____
____

Exercise	**Duration**

Total calories burned______

EXCESSIVE DRINKING IS DETRIMENTAL TO THE HEALTH OF MOST PEOPLE!

Monday	Breakast	Lunch	Dinner
	3 slices bacon	Grilled Jumbo Shrimp	4 ozs. pork roast
	1 raspberry muffin	Medium Salad w/dressing	Yams
	1 cup raspberries	½ cup salted s/flower seeds	Cauliflower
	6 ozs. pineapple j.	1 coffee/tea	Small green salad
	1 coffee/tea		8 ozs. apricot nectar

Snacks

4 tbsps. peanuts
½ cup peaches
1 vanilla yogurt
1 herbal tea

***Vegans replace dairy products with soy cheese and reconstituted non-dairy creamer. Every third day all weight managers should eat 1/2 cup beans, lentils, and other legumes.**

****Replace meat products with "chicken" (mushroom) tenders and meatballs (mushrooms). Full range of Quorn ® products is suggested for variety. You may also use soy products for protein intake if not a cancer survivor.**

Substitutions/notes/symptoms Indiscretions/distress/extra calories/etc. ____________________ ____________________ ____________________ ____________________ **Exercise Duration** **Total calories burned______**

BEANS AND OTHER LEGUMES IN COMBINATION WITH GRAINS PROVIDE SUPERIOR DIETARY PROTEIN.

Tuesday	Breakfast	Lunch	Dinner
	1 ½ ounce cereal	**6 ozs. Tuna salad w/ toast	**4 ozs. Beef
	*4 ozs. milk	Spinach Salad	Asparagus
	1 cup canned peaches	Fruit cocktail	Baked potato
	1 English muffin	Elderberry juice	Parsnips
	W/all fruit spread	Coffee/tea	
	Coffee/tea		

Snacks

1 oz. veggie chips
8 ozs. kefir
4 tbsps. filberts
1 herbal tea

***Vegans replace dairy products with soy cheese and reconstituted non-dairy creamer. Every third day all weight managers should eat 1/2 cup beans, lentils, and other legumes.**

**** Vegans/Vegetarians replace meat products with "chicken" (mushroom) tenders and meatballs (mushrooms). Full range of Quorn ® products is suggested for variety. You may also use soy products for protein intake if not a cancer survivor.**

Weigh-in: Wednesday

Cycle 13 (4 days)

Substitutions/notes/symptoms Indiscretions/distress/extra calories/etc.

____

____

____

____

Exercise Duration

Total calories burned______

DO I REALLY NEED VITAMINS IS LIKE ASKING DO I REALLY NEED INSURANCE!

Wednesday	Breakfast	Lunch	Dinner
	egg beaters® omelet scrambled with peppers/ onions /sour cream dollop	Turkey Salad	4-6 ozs. fish
	1 slice toast w/butter	Green salad	Zucchini
	Coffee/tea	½ cup pineapple	Carrots
		Coffee/tea	½ cup buttered pasta
		Raw carrot juice	

Snacks

1 oz. potato chips
1 oz. black-eyed peas
8 elderberry juice
½ cup canned/fresh apricots
1 herbal tea

***Vegans replace dairy products with soy cheese and non-dairy creamer reconstituted.**

****Replace meat products with "chicken" (mushroom) tenders and meatballs (mushrooms). Full range of Quorn ® products is suggested for variety. You may also use soy products for protein intake if not a cancer survivor.**

Substitutions/notes/symptoms
Indiscretions/distress/extra calories/etc.

____
____
____
____

Exercise	**Duration**

Total calories burned______

IF YOU THINK THE FOOD CHAIN IS AS HEALTHY TODAY AS IT WAS A DECADE OR SO AGO, ASK THE NUCLEAR SCIENTISTS AND FARMERS OF TODAY!

Thursday	**Breakfast**	**Lunch**	**Dinner**
	2 slices bacon	Shrimp Salad	4 ozs. pork
	1 blueberry muffin	Coleslaw	Peas
	1 cup kefir	Green Salad	Rice w/mushrooms
	Coffee/tea	Coffee/tea	Summer/Winter Squash

Snacks

8 ozs. carrot juice
1 cup strawberries
1 cup English walnuts
1 herbal tea

*Vegans replace dairy products with soy cheese and reconstituted non-dairy creamer. Every third day all weight managers should eat 1/2 cup beans, lentils, and other legumes.

**Replace meat products with "chicken" (mushroom) tenders and meatballs (mushrooms). Full range of Quorn ® products is suggested for variety. You may also use soy products for protein intake if not a cancer survivor.

Substitutions/notes/symptoms Indiscretions/distress/extra calories/etc.
____
____
____
____
Exercise Duration
Total calories burned______

IS IT BETTER BECAUSE IT IS FRESH? YES, IF IT IS PROPERLY CLEANED!

Friday	Breakfast	Lunch	Dinner
	2 slices "lite" toast	1 chef salad (chicken)	4 ozs. turkey
	1 pat butter	1 cup carrot juice	1 cup rice w/butter
	½ cup pears	1 cup blueberries	½ cup coleslaw
	½ cup ricotta/c.cheese	1 coffee/tea	8 ozs. cranberry juice
	1 coffee/tea		

Snacks

2 kiwi fruits
1 cup pineapple juice
1 cup English walnuts
1 herbal tea

*Vegans replace dairy products with soy cheese and reconstituted non-dairy creamer. Every third day all weight managers should eat 1/2 cup beans, lentils, and other legumes.

**Replace meat products with "chicken" (mushroom) tenders and meatballs (mushrooms). Full range of Quorn ® products is suggested for variety. You may also use soy products for protein intake if not a cancer survivor.

Substitutions/notes/symptoms Indiscretions/distress/extra calories/etc.	HAVE I DONE MY EXERCISE TODAY?
______________________________ ______________________________ ______________________________ __________________________ Exercise Duration ______________________________ Total calories burned______	

Saturday	Breakast	Lunch	Dinner
	1 ½ oz. cereal	4 ozs. chipped beef	4 ozs. fish
	* 4 ozs. milk	spinach salad	fiddlehead ferns
	1 cup blackberries	1 cup tangerine slices	Whole kernel corn
	1 English muffin	1 coffee/tea	Fresh parsnips
	1 coffee/tea		

Snacks

2 kiwi fruits
1 cup pineapple juice
1 cup English walnuts
1 herbal tea

*Vegans replace dairy products with soy cheese and reconstituted non-dairy creamer. Every third day all weight managers should eat 1/2 cup beans, lentils, and other legumes.

**Replace meat products with "chicken" (mushroom) tenders and meatballs (mushrooms). Full range of Quorn ® products is suggested for variety. You may also use soy products for protein intake if not a cancer survivor.

Cycle 14 (4 days)

Substitutions/notes/symptoms
Indiscretions/distress/extra calories/etc.
____
____
____
____

Exercise **Duration**

Total calories burned______

HAVE I DONE MY BONES A FAVOR BY USING SOME FORM OF WEIGHT TRAINING EXERCISE TODAY?

Sunday	Breakfast	Lunch	Dinner
	2 eggs	Turkey sandwich	½ Cornish hen
	1 slice "lite" toast	Caesar salad	Macaroni & Cheese
	1 cup strawberries	½ cup salted s/flower seeds	Broccoli rabe
	6 ozs. orange juice	1 coffee/tea	Small green salad
	1 coffee/tea		8 ozs. elderberry juice

Snacks

1 oz. pita chips
Celery/Parsley/Apple Juice
½ cup beans
Flavored water
1 herbal tea

***Vegans replace dairy products with soy cheese and reconstituted non-dairy creamer. Every third day all weight managers should eat 1/2 cup beans, lentils, and other legumes.**

****Replace meat products with "chicken" (mushroom) tenders and meatballs (mushrooms). Full range of Quorn ® products is suggested for variety. You may also use soy products for protein intake if not a cancer survivor.**

Substitutions/notes/symptoms
Indiscretions/distress/extra calories/etc.

____
____
____
____

Exercise Duration

Total calories burned______

EXCESSIVE DRINKING IS DETRIMENTAL TO THE HEALTH OF MOST PEOPLE!

Monday	**Breakast**	**Lunch**	**Dinner**
	3 slices bacon	Grilled Jumbo Shrimp	4 ozs. pork roast
	1 raspberry muffin	Medium Salad w/dressing	Yams
	1 cup raspberries	½ cup salted s/flower seeds	Cauliflower
	6 ozs. pineapple j.	1 coffee/tea	Small salad
	1 coffee/tea		8 ozs. apricot n.

Snacks

4 tbsps. peanuts
½ cup peaches
1 vanilla yogurt
1 herbal tea

***Vegans replace dairy products with soy cheese and reconstituted non-dairy creamer. Every third day all weight managers should eat 1/2 cup beans, lentils, and other legumes.**

****Replace meat products with "chicken" (mushroom) tenders and meatballs (mushrooms). Full range of Quorn ® products is suggested for variety. You may also use soy products for protein intake if not a cancer survivor.**

Substitutions/notes/symptoms Indiscretions/distress/extra calories/etc.

____

____

____

____

Exercise Duration

Total calories burned

BEANS AND OTHER LEGUMES IN COMBINATION WITH GRAINS PROVIDE SUPERIOR DIETARY PROTEIN.

Tuesday	Breakfast	Lunch	Dinner
	1 ½ ounce cereal	**6 ozs. Tuna salad/toast	**4 ozs. Beef
	*4 ozs. milk	Spinach Salad	Asparagus
	1 cup canned peaches	Fruit cocktail	Rice pasta
	1 English muffin	Elderberry juice	Parsnips
	W/all fruit spread	Coffee/tea	
	Coffee/tea		

Snacks

Veggie chips
8 ozs. kefir
4 tbsps. peanuts
1 herbal tea

***Vegans replace dairy products with soy cheese and reconstituted non-dairy creamer. Every third day all weight managers should eat 1/2 cup beans, lentils, and other legumes.**

**** Vegans/Vegetarians replace meat products with "chicken" (mushroom) tenders and meatballs (mushrooms). Full range of Quorn ® products is suggested for variety. You may also use soy products for protein intake if not a cancer survivor.**

Substitutions/notes/symptoms Indiscretions/distress/extra calories/etc.	**HAVE I DONE MY EXERCISE TODAY?**
______________________________ ______________________________ ______________________________ __________________________ **Exercise** **Duration** **Total calories burned______**	

Wednesday	**Breakfast**	**Lunch**	**Dinner**
	egg beaters® omelet scrambled with peppers/ onions /sour cream dollop	**Turkey Salad**	**4-6 ozs. fish**
		Green salad	**Zucchini**
		½ cup pineapple	**Carrots**
	1 slice toast w/butter	**Coffee/tea**	**½ cup buttered pasta**
	Coffee/tea	**Raw carrot juice**	

Snacks

2 kiwi fruits
1 cup pineapple juice
1 cup English walnuts
1 herbal tea

***Vegans replace dairy products with soy cheese and reconstituted non-dairy creamer. Every third day all weight managers should eat 1/2 cup beans, lentils, and other legumes.**

****Replace meat products with "chicken" (mushroom) tenders and meatballs (mushrooms). Full range of Quorn ® products is suggested for variety. You may also use soy products for protein intake if not a cancer survivor.**

Substitutions/notes/symptoms Indiscretions/distress/extra calories/etc.
____
____
____
____
Exercise **Duration**
Total calories burned______

HAVE I DONE MY BONES A FAVOR BY USING SOME FORM OF WEIGHT TRAINING EXERCISE?

Thursday	Breakfast	Lunch	Dinner

Snacks

1 oz. pita chips
Celery/Parsley/Apple Juice
½ cup beans
Flavored water
1 herbal tea

***Vegans replace dairy products with soy cheese and reconstituted non-dairy creamer. Every third day all weight managers should eat 1/2 cup beans, lentils, and other legumes.**

****Replace meat products with "chicken" (mushroom) tenders and meatballs (mushrooms). Full range of Quorn ® products is suggested for variety. You may also use soy products for protein intake if not a cancer survivor.**

Substitutions/notes/symptoms Indiscretions/distress/extra calories/etc.

____
____
____
____

Exercise Duration

Total calories burned

EXCESSIVE DRINKING IS DETRIMENTAL TO THE HEALTH OF MOST PEOPLE!

Friday	**Breakfast**	**Lunch**	**Dinner**

Snacks

4 tbsps. peanuts
½ cup peaches
1 vanilla yogurt
1 herbal tea

***Vegans replace dairy products with soy cheese and reconstituted non-dairy creamer. Every third day all weight managers should eat 1/2 cup beans, lentils, and other legumes.**

****Replace meat products with "chicken" (mushroom) tenders and meatballs (mushrooms). Full range of Quorn ® products is suggested for variety. You may also use soy products for protein intake if not a cancer survivor.**

Substitutions/notes/symptoms
Indiscretions/distress/extra calories/etc.

____
____
____
____

Exercise Duration

____

Total calories burned

BEANS AND OTHER LEGUMES IN COMBINATION WITH GRAINS PROVIDE SUPERIOR DIETARY PROTEIN.

Saturday	**Breakfast**	**Lunch**	**Dinner**

Snacks

1 oz. veggie chips
8 ozs. kefir
4 tbsps. peanuts
1 herbal tea

***Vegans replace dairy products with soy cheese and reconstituted non-dairy creamer. Every third day all weight managers should eat 1/2 cup beans, lentils, and other legumes.**

**** Vegans/Vegetarians replace meat products with "chicken" (mushroom) tenders and meatballs (mushrooms). Full range of Quorn ® products is suggested for variety. You may also use soy products for protein intake if not a cancer survivor.**

Substitutions/notes/symptoms Indiscretions/distress/extra calories/etc.

____
____
____
____
____

Exercise Duration

Total calories burned______

IS TURBINADO SUGAR BETTER THAN TABLE SUGAR? NO. THE ONLY REAL DIFFERENCE IS IN THE COLOR!

Sunday	Breakfast	Lunch	Dinner

Snacks

1 oz. potato chips
Celery/Parsley/Apple Juice
½ cup lentils
20-40 grapes
1 herbal tea

***Vegans replace dairy products with soy cheese and reconstituted non-dairy creamer. Every third day all weight managers should eat 1/2 cup beans, lentils, and other legumes.**

****Replace meat products with "chicken" (mushroom) tenders and meatballs (mushrooms). Full range of Quorn ® products is suggested for variety. You may also use soy products for protein intake if not a cancer survivor.**

Substitutions/notes/symptoms Indiscretions/distress/extra calories/etc.

____

____

____

____

Exercise Duration

Total calories burned______

ARE THERE ANY "LIVE CELLS" IN THE FOOD I ATE TODAY?

Monday Breakfast Lunch Dinner

Snacks

1 apple
1 oz. fried pork rinds
1blueberry yogurt
1 herbal tea

***Vegans replace dairy products with soy cheese and reconstituted non-dairy creamer. Every third day all weight managers should eat 1/2 cup beans, lentils, and other legumes.**

****Replace meat products with "chicken" (mushroom) tenders and meatballs (mushrooms). Full range of Quorn ® products is suggested for variety. You may also use soy products for protein intake if not a cancer survivor.**

Substitutions/notes/symptoms Indiscretions/distress/extra calories/etc.

____
____
____
____
____

Exercise Duration

Total calories burned______

WHAT HAVE I DONE FOR MY HEART TODAY?

Tuesday	**Breakfast**	**Lunch**	**Dinner**

Snacks

4 tbsps. walnuts
½ cup fruit cocktail
1 vanilla yogurt
1 herbal tea

***Vegans replace dairy products with soy cheese and reconstituted non-dairy creamer. Every third day all weight managers should eat 1/2 cup beans, lentils, and other legumes.**

****Replace meat products with "chicken" (mushroom) tenders and meatballs (mushrooms). Full range of Quorn ® products is suggested for variety. You may also use soy products for protein intake if not a cancer survivor.**

Substitutions/notes/symptoms Indiscretions/distress/extra calories/etc. ____________________ ____________________ ____________________ ____________________ **Exercise** **Duration** **Total calories burned______**

ARE MY SUPPLEMENTS COMPREHENSIVE AND IN CORRECT DOSAGES?

Wednesday	Breakfast	Lunch	Dinner

Snacks

4 tbsps. peanuts
1 orange
1 strawberry yogurt
1 herbal tea

***Vegans replace dairy products with soy cheese and reconstituted non-dairy creamer. Every third day all weight managers should eat 1/2 cup beans, lentils, and other legumes.**

****Replace meat products with "chicken" (mushroom) tenders and meatballs (mushrooms). Full range of Quorn ® products is suggested for variety. You may also use soy products for protein intake if not a cancer survivor.**

Substitutions/notes/symptoms **Indiscretions/distress/extra calories/etc.** ______________________________ ______________________________ ______________________________ ______________________________ **Exercise Duration** **Total calories burned______**

REMEMBER TO TAKE YOUR INDIVIDUALLY PLANNED SUPPLEMENTS EACH DAY!

Thursday	**Breakfast**	**Lunch**	**Dinner**

Snacks

½ cup beans/lentils
1 pear
1 banana
1 herbal tea

***Vegans replace dairy products with soy cheese and reconstituted non-dairy creamer. Every third day all weight managers should eat 1/2 cup beans, lentils, and other legumes.**

****Replace meat products with "chicken" (mushroom) tenders and meatballs (mushrooms). Full range of Quorn ® products is suggested for variety. You may also use soy products for protein intake if not a cancer survivor.**

Substitutions/notes/symptoms Indiscretions/distress/extra calories/etc.

____
____
____
____
____

Exercise Duration

Total calories burned______

HAVE I EATEN ANYTHING "LIVE" IN THE LAST FOUR DAYS?

Friday	Breakfast	Lunch	Dinner

Snacks

4 tbsps. filberts
½ cup mandarin orange slices
1 plain yogurt
1 herbal tea

***Vegans replace dairy products with soy cheese and reconstituted non-dairy creamer. Every third day all weight managers should eat 1/2 cup beans, lentils, and other legumes.**

****Replace meat products with "chicken" (mushroom) tenders and meatballs (mushrooms). Full range of Quorn ® products is suggested for variety. You may also use soy products for protein intake if not a cancer survivor.**

Substitutions/notes/symptoms
Indiscretions/distress/extra calories/etc.

____
____
____
____

Exercise Duration

Total calories burned______

IS IT POSSIBLE FOR ELECTROMAGNETIC ENERGY TO BE CREATED IN MY CELLS WITH "DEAD" FOOD

Saturday	**Breakfast**	**Lunch**	**Dinner**

Snacks

4 tbsps. peanuts
½ cup peaches
1 vanilla yogurt
1 herbal tea

***Vegans replace dairy products with soy cheese and reconstituted non-dairy creamer. Every third day all weight managers should eat 1/2 cup beans, lentils, and other legumes.**

****Replace meat products with "chicken" (mushroom) tenders and meatballs (mushrooms). Full range of Quorn ® products is suggested for variety. You may also use soy products for protein intake if not a cancer survivor.**

Substitutions/notes/symptoms Indiscretions/distress/extra calories/etc.

____

____

____

____

Exercise Duration

Total calories burned______

ARE MY BONES, MUSCLES, AND HEART ANY HEALTHIER BECAUSE I GAVE THEM SOME UNDIVIDED ATTENTION TODAY??

Sunday	**Breakfast**	**Lunch**	**Dinner**

Snacks

½ grapefruit
1 cup pineapple chunks
1 vanilla yogurt
1 oz. potato chips
1 herbal tea

***Vegans replace dairy products with soy cheese and reconstituted non-dairy creamer. Every third day all weight managers should eat 1/2 cup beans, lentils, and other legumes.**

****Replace meat products with "chicken" (mushroom) tenders and meatballs (mushrooms). Full range of Quorn ® products is suggested for variety. You may also use soy products for protein intake if not a cancer survivor.**

Substitutions/notes/symptoms Indiscretions/distress/extra calories/etc.

____

____

____

____

Exercise **Duration**

Total calories burned______

HOW MUCH OF A CHEMICAL ONSLAUGHT WAS PRESENT IN MY DIET AND ENVIRONMENT TODAY?

Monday	**Breakfast**	**Lunch**	**Dinner**

Snacks

½ peanut butter/all fruit sandwich on "lite"
1 cup lentils/beans
1 cup blackberries
8 ozs. strawberry kefir
1 herbal tea

***Vegans replace dairy products with soy cheese and reconstituted non-dairy creamer. Every third day all weight managers should eat 1/2 cup beans, lentils, and other legumes.**

****Replace meat products with "chicken" (mushroom) tenders and meatballs (mushrooms). Full range of Quorn ® products is suggested for variety. You may also use soy products for protein intake if not a cancer survivor.**

Substitutions/notes/symptoms Indiscretions/distress/extra calories/etc.

____
____
____
____

Exercise Duration

Total calories burned______

ARE THERE MYRIAD SUBSTANCES IN MY FOOD THAT I CAN'T EVEN PRONOUNCE?

Tuesday	**Breakfast**	**Lunch**	**Dinner**

Snacks

4 tbsps. cashews
1 oz. dried apricots
8 ozs. raspberry kefir
1 oz. fried pork rinds
1 herbal tea

***Vegans replace dairy products with soy cheese and reconstituted non-dairy creamer. Every third day all weight managers should eat 1/2 cup beans, lentils, and other legumes.**

****Replace meat products with "chicken" (mushroom) tenders and meatballs (mushrooms). Full range of Quorn ® products is suggested for variety. You may also use soy products for protein intake if not a cancer survivor.**

Substitutions/notes/symptoms Indiscretions/distress/extra calories/etc.

____

____

____

____

Exercise	Duration

Total calories burned______

BY HOW MUCH DID THE "LIVE" CELLS IN MY FOOD TODAY OUTWEIGH THE CHEMICAL AND "DEAD" CELLS ?

Wednesday	Breakfast	Lunch	Dinner

Snacks

1 oz. pita chips
Celery/Parsley/Apple Juice
5 tbsps. pumpkin seeds
Flavored water
1 herbal tea

***Vegans replace dairy products with soy cheese and reconstituted non-dairy creamer. Every third day all weight managers should eat 1/2 cup beans, lentils, and other legumes.**

****Replace meat products with "chicken" (mushroom) tenders and meatballs (mushrooms). Full range of Quorn ® products is suggested for variety. You may also use soy products for protein intake if not a cancer survivor.**

Substitutions/notes/symptoms Indiscretions/distress/extra calories/etc.

____

____

____

Exercise Duration

Total calories burned______

IS RICE BETTER THAN POTATOES? WHY?

Thursday	**Breakfast**	**Lunch**	**Dinner**

Snacks

½ cup lentils/beans
1 oz. veggie chips
8 ozs. peach kefir
4 tbsps. macadamia nuts
1 herbal tea

***Vegans replace dairy products with soy cheese and reconstituted non-dairy creamer. Every third day all weight managers should eat 1/2 cup beans, lentils, and other legumes.**

**** Vegans/Vegetarians replace meat products with "chicken" (mushroom) tenders and meatballs (mushrooms). Full range of Quorn ® products is suggested for variety. You may also use soy products for protein intake if not a cancer survivor.**

Substitutions/notes/symptoms
Indiscretions/distress/extra calories/etc.
____
____
____
____
____

Exercise **Duration**

Total calories burned______

DOES MY EXERCISE REGIMEN MATCH AND BURN THE NUMBER OF EXCESSIVE CALORIES I HAVE TAKEN IN DURING THE LAST FOUR DAYS?

Friday	**Breakfast**	**Lunch**	**Dinner**

Snacks

1 oz. potato chips
8 ozs. elderberry juice
½ cup canned/fresh apricots
1 herbal tea

***Vegans replace dairy products with soy cheese and non-dairy creamer reconstituted.**

****Replace meat products with "chicken" (mushroom) tenders and meatballs (mushrooms). Full range of Quorn ® products is suggested for variety. You may also use soy products for protein intake if not a cancer survivor.**

Substitutions/notes/symptoms Indiscretions/distress/extra calories/etc.

____

____

____

____

Exercise Duration

Total calories burned______

SHOULD I BURN LAST WEEK'S EXTRA CALORIES TODAY OR SHOULD I WAIT SIX MONTHS? ASK YOUR WAISTLINE!

Saturday	Breakfast	Lunch	Dinner

Snacks

1 oz. veggie chips
1 orange
20-40 seedless grapes
1 cup fresh cherries (frozen if not in season)
1 herbal tea

***Vegans replace dairy products with soy cheese and reconstituted non-dairy creamer. Every third day all weight managers should eat 1/2 cup beans, lentils, and other legumes.**

**** Vegans/Vegetarians replace meat products with "chicken" (mushroom) tenders and meatballs (mushrooms). Full range of Quorn ® products is suggested for variety. You may also use soy products for protein intake if not a cancer survivor.**

Substitutions/notes/symptoms Indiscretions/distress/extra calories/etc. _____________________________ _____________________________ _____________________________ _____________________________ **Exercise Duration** **Total calories burned______**

WAS THERE SOMETHING I ATE TODAY THAT DID NOT AGREE WITH ME?

Sunday	Breakfast	Lunch	Dinner

Snacks

4 tbsps. peanuts
1 cup watermelon slices
1 oz. potato chips
1 blueberry yogurt
1 herbal tea

***Vegans replace dairy products with soy cheese and reconstituted non-dairy creamer. Every third day all weight managers should eat 1/2 cup beans, lentils, and other legumes.**

****Replace meat products with "chicken" (mushroom) tenders and meatballs (mushrooms). Full range of Quorn ® products is suggested for variety. You may also use soy products for protein intake if not a cancer survivor.**

Substitutions/notes/symptoms Indiscretions/distress/extra calories/etc.

____
____
____
____
____

Exercise Duration

Total calories burned______

WHAT IS PROCRASTINATION?

Monday	**Breakfast**	**Lunch**	**Dinner**

Snacks

4 tbsps. English walnuts
½ cup beans/lentils
½ cup fruit cocktail
1 strawberry yogurt
1 herbal tea

***Vegans replace dairy products with soy cheese and reconstituted non-dairy creamer. Every third day all weight managers should eat 1/2 cup beans, lentils, and other legumes.**

****Replace meat products with "chicken" (mushroom) tenders and meatballs (mushrooms). Full range of Quorn ® products is suggested for variety. You may also use soy products for protein intake if not a cancer survivor.**

Substitutions/notes/symptoms
Indiscretions/distress/extra calories/etc.

____
____
____
____

Exercise **Duration**

Total calories burned______

DO I NEED LUTEIN?

Tuesday	**Breakfast**	**Lunch**	**Dinner**

Snacks

4 tbsps. macadamia nuts
1 apple
1 cup strawberries
1 vanilla yogurt
1 herbal tea

***Vegans replace dairy products with soy cheese and reconstituted non-dairy creamer. Every third day all weight managers should eat 1/2 cup beans, lentils, and other legumes.**

****Replace meat products with "chicken" (mushroom) tenders and meatballs (mushrooms). Full range of Quorn ® products is suggested for variety. You may also use soy products for protein intake if not a cancer survivor.**

Substitutions/notes/symptoms Indiscretions/distress/extra calories/etc.

____
____
____
____

Exercise	**Duration**

Total calories burned______

HOW MANY TIMES PER YEAR AM I SICK AND CAN IT BE AVOIDED?

Wednesday	**Breakfast**	**Lunch**	**Dinner**

Snacks

1 oz. veggie chips
½ cup raisins
1 vanilla yogurt
¼ cup lentils
1 herbal tea

***Vegans replace dairy products with soy cheese and reconstituted non-dairy creamer. Every third day all weight managers should eat 1/2 cup beans, lentils, and other legumes.**

****Replace meat products with "chicken" (mushroom) tenders and meatballs (mushrooms). Full range of Quorn ® products is suggested for variety. You may also use soy products for protein intake if not a cancer survivor.**

Substitutions/notes/symptoms
Indiscretions/distress/extra calories/etc.

____
____
____
____

Exercise Duration

Total calories burned______

WOULD A PEDOMETER INFORM ME AS TO WHETHER I AM REALLY A COUCH POTATO?

Thursday	Breakfast	Lunch	Dinner

Snacks

1 oz. veggie chips
8 ozs. raspberry kefir
4 tbsps. cashews
20-40 grapes
1 herbal tea

***Vegans replace dairy products with soy cheese and reconstituted non-dairy creamer. Every third day all weight managers should eat 1/2 cup beans, lentils, and other legumes.**

**** Vegans/Vegetarians replace meat products with "chicken" (mushroom) tenders and meatballs (mushrooms). Full range of Quorn ® products is suggested for variety. You may also use soy products for protein intake if not a cancer survivor.**

Substitutions/notes/symptoms
Indiscretions/distress/extra calories/etc.

____
____
____
____

Exercise Duration

Total calories burned______

EXCESSIVE DRINKING IS DETRIMENTAL TO THE HELP OF MOST PEOPLE!

Friday	**Breakfast**	**Lunch**	**Dinner**

Snacks

4 tbsps. black walnuts
½ cup peaches
1 vanilla yogurt
1 herbal tea

***Vegans replace dairy products with soy cheese and reconstituted non-dairy creamer. Every third day all weight managers should eat 1/2 cup beans, lentils, and other legumes.**

****Replace meat products with "chicken" (mushroom) tenders and meatballs (mushrooms). Full range of Quorn ® products is suggested for variety. You may also use soy products for protein intake if not a cancer survivor.**

Substitutions/notes/symptoms Indiscretions/distress/extra calories/etc.	DO I TAKE MEDICINES THAT ARE UNNECESSARY FOR MY HEALTH?
______________________________ ______________________________ ______________________________ ______________________________ ________	
Exercise **Duration**	
Total calories burned______	

Saturday Breakfast Lunch Dinner

Snacks

1 oz. English walnuts
20-40 grapes (any variety)
1 Orange
1 vanilla yogurt
1 herbal tea

***Vegans replace dairy products with soy cheese and reconstituted non-dairy creamer. Every third day all weight managers should eat 1/2 cup beans, lentils, and other legumes.**

****Replace meat products with "chicken" (mushroom) tenders and meatballs (mushrooms). Full range of Quorn ® products is suggested for variety. You may also use soy products for protein intake if not a cancer survivor.**

Substitutions/notes/symptoms Indiscretions/distress/extra calories/etc.

____
____
____
____

Exercise	**Duration**

Total calories burned______

DO I THINK A PILL SOLVES ALL PROBLEMS?

Sunday	**Breakfast**	**Lunch**	**Dinner**

Snacks

½ cup beans/lentils
20-40-grapes
½ cup peaches
1 vanilla yogurt
1 herbal tea

***Vegans replace dairy products with soy cheese and reconstituted non-dairy creamer. Every third day all weight managers should eat 1/2 cup beans, lentils, and other legumes.**

****Replace meat products with "chicken" (mushroom) tenders and meatballs (mushrooms). Full range of Quorn ® products is suggested for variety. You may also use soy products for protein intake if not a cancer survivor.**

Substitutions/notes/symptoms
Indiscretions/distress/extra calories/etc.

____
____
____
____

Exercise **Duration**

Total calories burned______

HAVE I CHANGED MY WAY OF THINKING ABOUT FOOD?

Monday	**Breakfast**	**Lunch**	**Dinner**

Snacks

4 tbsps. peanuts
½ cup peaches
1 vanilla yogurt
1 herbal tea

***Vegans replace dairy products with soy cheese and reconstituted non-dairy creamer. Every third day all weight managers should eat 1/2 cup beans, lentils, and other legumes.**

****Replace meat products with "chicken" (mushroom) tenders and meatballs (mushrooms). Full range of Quorn ® products is suggested for variety. You may also use soy products for protein intake if not a cancer survivor.**

Substitutions/notes/symptoms
Indiscretions/distress/extra calories/etc.

____
____
____
____

Exercise Duration

Total calories burned______

FOOD IS THE FUNDAMENTAL MEANS OF EXISTENCE. LOVE, JOY, AND PEACE ARE BYPRODUCTS OF GOOD FOOD AND EXERCISE!

Tuesday	Breakfast	Lunch	Dinner

Snacks

1 oz. veggie chips
8 ozs. kefir
4 tbsps. peanuts
1 herbal tea

***Vegans replace dairy products with soy cheese and reconstituted non-dairy creamer. Every third day all weight managers should eat 1/2 cup beans, lentils, and other legumes.**

**** Vegans/Vegetarians replace meat products with "chicken" (mushroom) tenders and meatballs (mushrooms). Full range of Quorn ® products is suggested for variety. You may also use soy products for protein intake if not a cancer survivor.**

Substitutions/notes/symptoms Indiscretions/distress/extra calories/etc.
____
____
____
____
Exercise **Duration**
Total calories burned______

DID I STRETCH AND RELEASE ENERGY-GIVING GLUCOSE FROM MY MUSCLES TODAY?

Wednesday	Breakfast	Lunch	Dinner

Snacks

1 oz. potato chips
8 ozs. elderberry juice
½ cup canned/fresh apricots
1 herbal tea

***Vegans replace dairy products with soy cheese and non-dairy creamer reconstituted.**

****Replace meat products with "chicken" (mushroom) tenders and meatballs (mushrooms). Full range of Quorn ® products is suggested for variety. You may also use soy products for protein intake if not a cancer survivor.**

Substitutions/notes/symptoms
Indiscretions/distress/extra calories/etc.

____
____
____
____

Exercise Duration

Total calories burned______

DOES *LIVE* FOOD GIVE LIFE?

YOU BET!!!!

Thursday	Breakfast	Lunch	Dinner

Snacks

1 oz. pita chips
Celery/Parsley/Apple Juice
5 tbsps. pumpkin seeds
Flavored water
1 herbal tea

***Vegans replace dairy products with soy cheese and reconstituted non-dairy creamer. Every third day all weight managers should eat 1/2 cup beans, lentils, and other legumes.**

****Replace meat products with "chicken" (mushroom) tenders and meatballs (mushrooms). Full range of Quorn ® products is suggested for variety. You may also use soy products for protein intake if not a cancer survivor.**

Substitutions/notes/symptoms
Indiscretions/distress/extra calories/etc.

____
____
____
____

Exercise Duration

Total calories burned______

I CAN BE THE WEIGHT I WANT TO BE BY CAREFULLY MANAGING WHAT I PUT IN MY MOUTH!

Friday	**Breakfast**	**Lunch**	**Dinner**

Snacks

1 oz. potato chips
½ cup beans/lentils
8 elderberry juice
½ cup canned/fresh apricots
1 herbal tea

***Vegans replace dairy products with soy cheese and non-dairy creamer reconstituted.**

****Replace meat products with "chicken" (mushroom) tenders and meatballs (mushrooms). Full range of Quorn ® products is suggested for variety. You may also use soy products for protein intake if not a cancer survivor.**

Substitutions/notes/symptoms Indiscretions/distress/extra calories/etc.

____
____
____
____

Exercise Duration

Total calories burned______

WEIGHT AND AGE ARE NUMBERS MANIPULABLE BY WHAT I PUT IN MY MOUTH!

Saturday	**Breakfast**	**Lunch**	**Dinner**

Snacks

1 oz. veggie chips
½ cup raisins
1 vanilla yogurt
1 herbal tea

***Vegans replace dairy products with soy cheese and reconstituted non-dairy creamer. Every third day all weight managers should eat 1/2 cup beans, lentils, and other legumes.**

****Replace meat products with "chicken" (mushroom) tenders and meatballs (mushrooms). Full range of Quorn ® products is suggested for variety. You may also use soy products for protein intake if not a cancer survivor.**

Substitutions/notes/symptoms Indiscretions/distress/extra calories/etc.

____

____

____

____

Exercise Duration

Total calories burned______

HOW ATTRACTIVE AM I AT MY PRESENT WEIGHT?

Sunday	**Breakfast**	**Lunch**	**Dinner**

Snacks

4 tbsps. peanuts
½ cup fruit cocktail
8 ozs. peach kefir
1 tangerine
1 herbal tea

***Vegans replace dairy products with soy cheese and reconstituted non-dairy creamer. Every third day all weight managers should eat 1/2 cup beans, lentils, and other legumes.**

****Replace meat products with "chicken" (mushroom) tenders and meatballs (mushrooms). Full range of Quorn ® products is suggested for variety. You may also use soy products for protein intake if not a cancer survivor.**

Substitutions/notes/symptoms
Indiscretions/distress/extra calories/etc.

____
____
____
____

Exercise Duration

Total calories burned______

DO I THINK A PILL SOLVES ALL PROBLEMS?

Monday	**Breakfast**	**Lunch**	**Dinner**

Snacks

8 ozs. carrot juice
1 cup strawberries
1 oz. fried pork rinds
1 cup English walnuts
1 herbal tea

***Vegans replace dairy products with soy cheese and reconstituted non-dairy creamer. Every third day all weight managers should eat 1/2 cup beans, lentils, and other legumes.**

****Replace meat products with "chicken" (mushroom) tenders and meatballs (mushrooms). Full range of Quorn ® products is suggested for variety. You may also use soy products for protein intake if not a cancer survivor.**

Substitutions/notes/symptoms
Indiscretions/distress/extra calories/etc.

____
____
____
____

Exercise Duration

Total calories burned______

HAVE I CHANGED MY WAY OF THINKING ABOUT FOOD?

Tuesday	**Breakfast**	**Lunch**	**Dinner**

Snacks

1 oz. pita chips
Celery/Parsley/Apple Juice
5 tbsps. pumpkin seeds
Flavored water
1 herbal tea

***Vegans replace dairy products with soy cheese and reconstituted non-dairy creamer. Every third day all weight managers should eat 1/2 cup beans, lentils, and other legumes.**

****Replace meat products with “chicken” (mushroom) tenders and meatballs (mushrooms). Full range of Quorn ® products is suggested for variety. You may also use soy products for protein intake if not a cancer survivor.**

Substitutions/notes/symptoms Indiscretions/distress/extra calories/etc.

____
____
____
____

Exercise Duration

Total calories burned______

FOOD IS THE FUNDAMENTAL MEANS OF EXISTENCE. LOVE, JOY, AND PEACE ARE BYPRODUCTS OF GOOD FOOD AND EXERCISE!

Wednesday	Breakfast	Lunch	Dinner

Snacks

½ cup pinto beans
½ cup blackberries
1 raspberry yogurt
1 herbal tea

***Vegans replace dairy products with soy cheese and reconstituted non-dairy creamer. Every third day all weight managers should eat 1/2 cup beans, lentils, and other legumes.**

****Replace meat products with "chicken" (mushroom) tenders and meatballs (mushrooms). Full range of Quorn ® products is suggested for variety. You may also use soy products for protein intake if not a cancer survivor.**

Substitutions/notes/symptoms Indiscretions/distress/extra calories/etc.

____
____
____
____

Exercise Duration

Total calories burned______

SHOULD MY NUTRITIONAL THUMBPRINT INCLUDE THE USE OF CARBOHYDRATES?

BY ALL MEANS!!!!!

Thursday	**Breakfast**	**Lunch**	**Dinner**

Snacks

4 tbsps. filberts
½ grapefruit
1 vanilla yogurt
20-40 grapes
1 herbal tea

***Vegans replace dairy products with soy cheese and reconstituted non-dairy creamer. Every third day all weight managers should eat 1/2 cup beans, lentils, and other legumes.**

****Replace meat products with "chicken" (mushroom) tenders and meatballs (mushrooms). Full range of Quorn ® products is suggested for variety. You may also use soy products for protein intake if not a cancer survivor.**

Substitutions/notes/symptoms
Indiscretions/distress/extra calories/etc.

____
____
____
____

Exercise Duration

Total calories burned______

ARE THERE ANY MIRACLES LEFT?

EXERCISE IS A MIRACLE!

Friday	Breakfast	Lunch	Dinner

Snacks

4 tbsps. English walnuts
½ cup peaches
8 ozs. peach kefir
1 cup blueberries
1 herbal tea

***Vegans replace dairy products with soy cheese and reconstituted non-dairy creamer. Every third day all weight managers should eat 1/2 cup beans, lentils, and other legumes.**

****Replace meat products with "chicken" (mushroom) tenders and meatballs (mushrooms). Full range of Quorn ® products is suggested for variety. You may also use soy products for protein intake if not a cancer survivor.**

Substitutions/notes/symptoms Indiscretions/distress/extra calories/etc.

____

____

____

____

Exercise	**Duration**

Total calories burned______

I CAN BE THE WEIGHT I WANT TO BE BY CAREFULLY MANAGING WHAT I PUT IN MY MOUTH!

Saturday	**Breakfast**	**Lunch**	**Dinner**

Snacks

½ cup beans (any variety)
½ cup peaches
1 strawberry yogurt
1 apple
1 herbal tea

***Vegans replace dairy products with soy cheese and reconstituted non-dairy creamer. Every third day all weight managers should eat 1/2 cup beans, lentils, and other legumes.**

****Replace meat products with "chicken" (mushroom) tenders and meatballs (mushrooms). Full range of Quorn ® products is suggested for variety. You may also use soy products for protein intake if not a cancer survivor.**

Substitutions/notes/symptoms
Indiscretions/distress/extra calories/etc.

____

____

____

____

Exercise **Duration**

Total calories burned______

WEIGHT AND AGE ARE NUMBERS MANIPULABLE BY WHAT I PUT IN MY MOUTH!

Sunday	**Breakfast**	**Lunch**	**Dinner**

Snacks

1 oz. pita chips
Celery/Parsley/Apple Juice
5 tbsps. pumpkin seeds
Flavored water
1 herbal tea

***Vegans replace dairy products with soy cheese and reconstituted non-dairy creamer. Every third day all weight managers should eat 1/2 cup beans, lentils, and other legumes.**

****Replace meat products with "chicken" (mushroom) tenders and meatballs (mushrooms). Full range of Quorn ® products is suggested for variety. You may also use soy products for protein intake if not a cancer survivor.**

Substitutions/notes/symptoms Indiscretions/distress/extra calories/etc.

____

____

____

____

Exercise Duration

Total calories burned______

HOW ATTRACTIVE AM I AT MY PRESENT WEIGHT?

Monday	Breakfast	Lunch	Dinner

Snacks

1 orange
½ cup beans/lentils
1 oz. mixed nuts
1 vanilla yogurt
1 herbal tea

***Vegans replace dairy products with soy cheese and reconstituted non-dairy creamer. Every third day all weight managers should eat 1/2 cup beans, lentils, and other legumes.**

****Replace meat products with "chicken" (mushroom) tenders and meatballs (mushrooms). Full range of Quorn ® products is suggested for variety. You may also use soy products for protein intake if not a cancer survivor.**

Substitutions/notes/symptoms Indiscretions/distress/extra calories/etc.

____
____
____
____

Exercise	**Duration**

Total calories burned______

DO I THINK A PILL SOLVES ALL PROBLEMS?

Tuesday	**Breakfast**	**Lunch**	**Dinner**

<u>Snacks</u>

1 oz. pita chips
Celery/Parsley/Apple Juice
1 cup cantaloupe
Flavored water
1 herbal tea

***Vegans replace dairy products with soy cheese and reconstituted non-dairy creamer. Every third day all weight managers should eat 1/2 cup beans, lentils, and other legumes.**

****Replace meat products with "chicken" (mushroom) tenders and meatballs (mushrooms). Full range of Quorn ® products is suggested for variety. You may also use soy products for protein intake if not a cancer survivor.**

Substitutions/notes/symptoms Indiscretions/distress/extra calories/etc.

____

____

____

____

Exercise Duration

Total calories burned______

HAVE I CHANGED MY WAY OF THINKING ABOUT FOOD?

Wednesday	**Breakfast**	**Lunch**	**Dinner**

Snacks

1 oz. pita chips
Grapefruit Juice
Trail mix (almonds, dried papaya, dried cranberries, raisins, etc.)
Flavored water
1 herbal tea

***Vegans replace dairy products with soy cheese and reconstituted non-dairy creamer. Every third day all weight managers should eat 1/2 cup beans, lentils, and other legumes.**

****Replace meat products with "chicken" (mushroom) tenders and meatballs (mushrooms). Full range of Quorn ® products is suggested for variety. You may also use soy products for protein intake if not a cancer survivor.**

Substitutions/notes/symptoms Indiscretions/distress/extra calories/etc.

____

____

____

____

Exercise Duration

Total calories burned______

FOOD IS THE FUNDAMENTAL MEANS OF EXISTENCE. LOVE, JOY, AND PEACE ARE BYPRODUCTS OF GOOD FOOD AND EXERCISE!

Thursday	**Breakfast**	**Lunch**	**Dinner**

Snacks

½ peanut butter/all fruit spread sandwich on "lite" bread
½ cup fruit cocktail
8 ozs. peach kefir
1 hard-boiled egg
1 herbal tea

***Vegans replace dairy products with soy cheese and reconstituted non-dairy creamer. Every third day all weight managers should eat 1/2 cup beans, lentils, and other legumes.**

****Replace meat products with "chicken" (mushroom) tenders and meatballs (mushrooms). Full range of Quorn ® products is suggested for variety. You may also use soy products for protein intake if not a cancer survivor.**

Substitutions/notes/symptoms
Indiscretions/distress/extra calories/etc.

____
____
____
____

Exercise Duration

Total calories burned______

HAVE I DONE MY EXERCISE TODAY?

Friday	**Breakfast**	**Lunch**	**Dinner**

Snacks

1 oz. veggie chips
8 ozs. kefir
4 tbsps. macadamia nuts
1 herbal tea

***Vegans replace dairy products with soy cheese and reconstituted non-dairy creamer. Every third day all weight managers should eat 1/2 cup beans, lentils, and other legumes.**

**** Vegans/Vegetarians replace meat products with "chicken" (mushroom) tenders and meatballs (mushrooms). Full range of Quorn ® products is suggested for variety. You may also use soy products for protein intake if not a cancer survivor.**

Substitutions/notes/symptoms
Indiscretions/distress/extra calories/etc.

____
____
____
____

Exercise Duration

Total calories burned______

SMOKING IS DETRIMENTAL TO THE HEALTH OF MOST PEOPLE!

Saturday	**Breakfast**	**Lunch**	**Dinner**

Snacks

1 apple
2 kiwi fruits
½ cup beans (any variety)
8 ozs. kefir (plain)
1 herbal or green tea

***Vegans replace dairy products with soy cheese and reconstituted non-dairy creamer. Every third day all weight managers should eat 1/2 cup beans, lentils, and other legumes.**

****Replace meat products with "chicken" (mushroom) tenders and meatballs (mushrooms). Full range of Quorn ® products is suggested for variety. You may also use soy products for protein intake if not a cancer survivor.**

Substitutions/notes/symptoms
Indiscretions/distress/extra calories/etc.
____
____
____
____

Exercise Duration

Total calories burned______

I CAN BE THE WEIGHT I WANT TO BE BY CAREFULLY MANAGING WHAT I PUT IN MY MOUTH!

***YES*!!!!!!!!**

Sunday	**Breakfast**	**Lunch**	**Dinner**

Snacks

4 tbsps. macadamia nuts
1 cup blueberries
1 vanilla yogurt
1 herbal tea

***Vegans replace dairy products with soy cheese and reconstituted non-dairy creamer. Every third day all weight managers should eat 1/2 cup beans, lentils, and other legumes.**

****Replace meat products with "chicken" (mushroom) tenders and meatballs (mushrooms). Full range of Quorn ® products is suggested for variety. You may also use soy products for protein intake if not a cancer survivor.**

Substitutions/notes/symptoms Indiscretions/distress/extra calories/etc. ____________________________ ____________________________ ____________________________ ____________________________ **Exercise Duration** **Total calories burned______**

WEIGHT AND AGE ARE NUMBERS MANIPULABLE BY WHAT I PUT IN MY MOUTH!

Monday	Breakfast	Lunch	Dinner

Snacks

1 oz. potato chips
8 ozs. elderberry juice
½ cup canned/fresh apricots
1 herbal tea

***Vegans replace dairy products with soy cheese and reconstituted non-dairy creamer. Every third day all weight managers should eat 1/2 cup beans, lentils, and other legumes.**

****Replace meat products with "chicken" (mushroom) tenders and meatballs (mushrooms). Full range of Quorn ® products is suggested for variety. You may also use soy products for protein intake if not a cancer survivor.**

Substitutions/notes/symptoms Indiscretions/distress/extra calories/etc.

____

____

____

____

Exercise **Duration**

Total calories burned______

HOW ATTRACTIVE AM I AT MY PRESENT WEIGHT?

Tuesday	**Breakfast**	**Lunch**	**Dinner**

Snacks

4 tbsps. peanuts
½ cup peaches
1 vanilla yogurt
1 herbal tea

***Vegans replace dairy products with soy cheese and reconstituted non-dairy creamer. Every third day all weight managers should eat 1/2 cup beans, lentils, and other legumes.**

****Replace meat products with "chicken" (mushroom) tenders and meatballs (mushrooms). Full range of Quorn ® products is suggested for variety. You may also use soy products for protein intake if not a cancer survivor.**

Substitutions/notes/symptoms Indiscretions/distress/extra calories/etc.
____
____
____
____
Exercise **Duration**
Total calories burned______

DO I THINK A PILL SOLVES ALL PROBLEMS?

Wednesday	Breakfast	Lunch	Dinner

Snacks

2 oranges
1 raspberry yogurt
½ cup beans (any variety)
1 oz. fried pork rinds
1 herbal tea

***Vegans replace dairy products with soy cheese and reconstituted non-dairy creamer. Every third day all weight managers should eat 1/2 cup beans, lentils, and other legumes.**

****Replace meat products with "chicken" (mushroom) tenders and meatballs (mushrooms). Full range of Quorn ® products is suggested for variety. You may also use soy products for protein intake if not a cancer survivor.**

Substitutions/notes/symptoms Indiscretions/distress/extra calories/etc.

____

____

____

____

Exercise Duration

____

Total calories burned______

HAVE I CHANGED MY WAY OF THINKING ABOUT FOOD?

Thursday	**Breakfast**	**Lunch**	**Dinner**

Snacks

8 ozs. carrot juice
1 cup strawberries
1 cup English walnuts
1 herbal tea

***Vegans replace dairy products with soy cheese and reconstituted non-dairy creamer. Every third day all weight managers should eat 1/2 cup beans, lentils, and other legumes.**

****Replace meat products with "chicken" (mushroom) tenders and meatballs (mushrooms). Full range of Quorn ® products is suggested for variety. You may also use soy products for protein intake if not a cancer survivor.**

Substitutions/notes/symptoms
Indiscretions/distress/extra calories/etc.

____
____
____
____

Exercise Duration

Total calories burned______

FOOD IS THE FUNDAMENTAL MEANS OF EXISTENCE. LOVE, JOY, AND PEACE ARE BYPRODUCTS OF GOOD FOOD AND EXERCISE!

Friday	**Breakfast**	**Lunch**	**Dinner**

Snacks

2 pears
2 shortbread cookies
1 herbal tea
1 vanilla yogurt

***Vegans replace dairy products with soy cheese and reconstituted non-dairy creamer. Every third day all weight managers should eat 1/2 cup beans, lentils, and other legumes.**

****Replace meat products with "chicken" (mushroom) tenders and meatballs (mushrooms). Full range of Quorn ® products is suggested for variety. You may also use soy products for protein intake if not a cancer survivor.**

Substitutions/notes/symptoms
Indiscretions/distress/extra calories/etc.

____
____
____
____

Exercise Duration

Total calories burned______

HOW IMPORTANT IS HEALTH? WITHOUT IT YOU HAVE NOTHING

Saturday	**Breakfast**	**Lunch**	**Dinner**

Snacks

1 oz. cashews
1 glass carrot juice
5 tbsps. pumpkin seeds
Flavored water
1 herbal tea

***Vegans replace dairy products with soy cheese and reconstituted non-dairy creamer. Every third day all weight managers should eat 1/2 cup beans, lentils, and other legumes.**

****Replace meat products with "chicken" (mushroom) tenders and meatballs (mushrooms). Full range of Quorn ® products is suggested for variety. You may also use soy products for protein intake if not a cancer survivor.**

Substitutions/notes/symptoms Indiscretions/distress/extra calories/etc.

____
____
____
____

Exercise Duration

Total calories burned______

HAVE I DONE MY BONES A FAVOR BY USING SOME FORM OF WEIGHT TRAINING EXERCISE?

Sunday	**Breakfast**	**Lunch**	**Dinner**

Snacks

½ cup pineapple
½ cup lentils (any variety)
1 oz. potato chips
1 vanilla yogurt
1 herbal tea

***Vegans replace dairy products with soy cheese and reconstituted non-dairy creamer. Every third day all weight managers should eat 1/2 cup beans, lentils, and other legumes.**

****Replace meat products with "chicken" (mushroom) tenders and meatballs (mushrooms). Full range of Quorn ® products is suggested for variety. You may also use soy products for protein intake if not a cancer survivor.**

Substitutions/notes/symptoms
Indiscretions/distress/extra calories/etc.

____
____
____
____

Exercise Duration

Total calories burned______

I CAN BE THE WEIGHT I WANT TO BE BY CAREFULLY MANAGING WHAT I PUT IN MY MOUTH!

Monday	**Breakfast**	**Lunch**	**Dinner**

Snacks

4 tbsps. filberts
1 fresh pear
1 strawberry yogurt
1 herbal tea

***Vegans replace dairy products with soy cheese and reconstituted non-dairy creamer. Every third day all weight managers should eat 1/2 cup beans, lentils, and other legumes.**

****Replace meat products with "chicken" (mushroom) tenders and meatballs (mushrooms). Full range of Quorn ® products is suggested for variety. You may also use soy products for protein intake if not a cancer survivor.**

Substitutions/notes/symptoms
Indiscretions/distress/extra calories/etc.

____
____
____
____

Exercise **Duration**

____

Total Calories Burned___________

WEIGHT AND AGE ARE NUMBERS MANIPULABLE BY WHAT I PUT IN MY MOUTH!

Tuesday	**Breakfast**	**Lunch**	**Dinner**

Snacks

1 oz. potato chips
8 ozs. elderberry juice
½ cup canned/fresh apricots
1 herbal tea

***Vegans replace dairy products with soy cheese and reconstituted non-dairy creamer. Every third day all weight managers should eat 1/2 cup beans, lentils, and other legumes.**

****Replace meat products with "chicken" (mushroom) tenders and meatballs (mushrooms). Full range of Quorn ® products is suggested for variety. You may also use soy products for protein intake if not a cancer survivor.**

Substitutions/notes/symptoms
Indiscretions/distress/extra calories/etc.

____
____
____
____

Exercise	**Duration**

Total calories burned______

IS IT POSSIBLE FOR ELECTROMAGNETIC ENERGY TO BE CREATED IN MY CELLS WITH "DEAD" FOOD?

Wednesday	**Breakfast**	**Lunch**	**Dinner**

Snacks

4 tbsps. peanuts
½ cup peaches
1 vanilla yogurt
1 herbal tea

***Vegans replace dairy products with soy cheese and reconstituted non-dairy creamer. Every third day all weight managers should eat 1/2 cup beans, lentils, and other legumes.**

****Replace meat products with "chicken" (mushroom) tenders and meatballs (mushrooms). Full range of Quorn ® products is suggested for variety. You may also use soy products for protein intake if not a cancer survivor.**

Substitutions/notes/symptoms Indiscretions/distress/extra calories/etc.

____
____
____
____
____

Exercise **Duration**

Total calories burned______

ASKING IF I NEED TO TAKE VITAMINS IS LIKE ASKING IF I NEED INSURANCE.

Thursday	**Breakfast**	**Lunch**	**Dinner**

Snacks

1 oz. veggie chips
8 ozs. kefir
4 tbsps. peanuts
1 herbal tea

***Vegans replace dairy products with soy cheese and reconstituted non-dairy creamer. Every third day all weight managers should eat 1/2 cup beans, lentils, and other legumes.**

**** Vegans/Vegetarians replace meat products with "chicken" (mushroom) tenders and meatballs (mushrooms). Full range of Quorn ® products is suggested for variety. You may also use soy products for protein intake if not a cancer survivor.**

Substitutions/notes/symptoms
Indiscretions/distress/extra calories/etc.

____
____
____
____
____

Exercise **Duration**

Total calories burned______

HAVE I CHANGED MY WAY OF THINKING ABOUT FOOD?

Friday	**Breakfast**	**Lunch**	**Dinner**

Snacks

8 ozs. carrot juice
½ cup beans/lentils
1 cup strawberries
1 cup English walnuts
1 herbal tea

***Vegans replace dairy products with soy cheese and reconstituted non-dairy creamer. Every third day all weight managers should eat 1/2 cup beans, lentils, and other legumes.**

****Replace meat products with "chicken" (mushroom) tenders and meatballs (mushrooms). Full range of Quorn ® products is suggested for variety. You may also use soy products for protein intake if not a cancer survivor.**

Substitutions/notes/symptoms
Indiscretions/distress/extra calories/etc.

____
____
____
____

Exercise Duration

Total calories burned______

FOOD IS THE FUNDAMENTAL MEANS OF EXISTENCE. LOVE, JOY, AND PEACE ARE BYPRODUCTS OF GOOD FOOD AND EXERCISE!

Saturday	**Breakfast**	**Lunch**	**Dinner**

Snacks

2 kiwi fruits
1 cup strawberries/blueberries
8 ozs. raspberry kefir
½ cup lentils (any variety)
1 herbal tea

***Vegans replace dairy products with soy cheese and reconstituted non-dairy creamer. Every third day all weight managers should eat 1/2 cup beans, lentils, and other legumes.**

****Replace meat products with "chicken" (mushroom) tenders and meatballs (mushrooms). Full range of Quorn ® products is suggested for variety. You may also use soy products for protein intake if not a cancer survivor.**

Substitutions/notes/symptoms Indiscretions/distress/extra calories/etc.

____
____
____
____

Exercise Duration

Total calories burned______

IF VITAMINS DON'T HELP ANYONE, TAKEN AS DIRECTED—ARE THEY LIKELY TO HARM ANYONE?

Sunday	**Breakfast**	**Lunch**	**Dinner**

Snacks

1 orange
1 cup strawberries
8 ozs. carrot juice
½ cup lentils
1 herbal tea

***Vegans replace dairy products with soy cheese and reconstituted non-dairy creamer. Every third day all weight managers should eat 1/2 cup beans, lentils, and other legumes.**

****Replace meat products with "chicken" (mushroom) tenders and meatballs (mushrooms). Full range of Quorn ® products is suggested for variety. You may also use soy products for protein intake if not a cancer survivor.**

Substitutions/notes/symptoms Indiscretions/distress/extra calories/etc.

____
____
____
____

Exercise	**Duration**

Total calories burned______

IF YOU THINK THE FOOD CHAIN IS AS HEALTHY TODAY AS IT WAS A DECADE OR SO AGO, ASK THE NUCLEAR SCIENTISTS AND FARMERS OF TODAY!

Monday	**Breakfast**	**Lunch**	**Dinner**

Snacks

1 oz. pita chips
Celery/Parsley/Apple Juice
5 tbsps. pumpkin seeds
Flavored water
1 herbal tea

***Vegans replace dairy products with soy cheese and reconstituted non-dairy creamer. Every third day all weight managers should eat 1/2 cup beans, lentils, and other legumes.**

****Replace meat products with "chicken" (mushroom) tenders and meatballs (mushrooms). Full range of Quorn ® products is suggested for variety. You may also use soy products for protein intake if not a cancer survivor.**

Substitutions/notes/symptoms
Indiscretions/distress/extra calories/etc.

____
____
____
____

Exercise Duration

Total calories burned______

IS IT POSSIBLE FOR ELECTROMAGNETIC ENERGY TO BE CREATED IN MY CELLS WITH "DEAD" FOOD

Tuesday	**Breakfast**	**Lunch**	**Dinner**

Snacks

8 ozs. carrot juice
1 cup strawberries
1 cup English walnuts
1 herbal tea

***Vegans replace dairy products with soy cheese and reconstituted non-dairy creamer. Every third day all weight managers should eat 1/2 cup beans, lentils, and other legumes.**

****Replace meat products with "chicken" (mushroom) tenders and meatballs (mushrooms). Full range of Quorn ® products is suggested for variety. You may also use soy products for protein intake if not a cancer survivor.**

Substitutions/notes/symptoms
Indiscretions/distress/extra calories/etc.

____

____

____

____

Exercise Duration

Total calories burned______

WEIGHT AND AGE ARE NUMBERS MANIPULABLE BY WHAT I PUT IN MY MOUTH!

Wednesday	Breakfast	Lunch	Dinner

Snacks

4 tbsps. walnuts
½ cup mandarin orange slices
1 plain yogurt
½ cup beans (any variety)
1 herbal tea

***Vegans replace dairy products with soy cheese and reconstituted non-dairy creamer. Every third day all weight managers should eat 1/2 cup beans, lentils, and other legumes.**

****Replace meat products with "chicken" (mushroom) tenders and meatballs (mushrooms). Full range of Quorn ® products is suggested for variety. You may also use soy products for protein intake if not a cancer survivor.**

Substitutions/notes/symptoms
Indiscretions/distress/extra calories/etc.

____
____
____
____

Exercise **Duration**

Total calories burned______

HOW ATTRACTIVE AM I AT MY PRESENT WEIGHT?

Thursday	**Breakfast**	**Lunch**	**Dinner**

Snacks

4 tbsps. peanuts
½ cup peaches
1 vanilla yogurt
1 herbal tea

***Vegans replace dairy products with soy cheese and reconstituted non-dairy creamer. Every third day all weight managers should eat 1/2 cup beans, lentils, and other legumes.**

****Replace meat products with "chicken" (mushroom) tenders and meatballs (mushrooms). Full range of Quorn ® products is suggested for variety. You may also use soy products for protein intake if not a cancer survivor.**

Substitutions/notes/symptoms
Indiscretions/distress/extra calories/etc.

____

____

____

____

Exercise	Duration

Total calories burned______

IS IT POSSIBLE FOR ELECTROMAGNETIC ENERGY TO BE CREATED IN MY CELLS WITH "DEAD" FOOD

Friday	Breakfast	Lunch	Dinner

Snacks

4 tbsps. mixed nuts
1 fresh peach
1 yogurt
½ cup Rice Dream ® (any flavor)
1 herbal tea

***Vegans replace dairy products with soy cheese and reconstituted non-dairy creamer. Every third day all weight managers should eat 1/2 cup beans, lentils, and other legumes.**

****Replace meat products with "chicken" (mushroom) tenders and meatballs (mushrooms). Full range of Quorn ® products is suggested for variety. You may also use soy products for protein intake if not a cancer survivor.**

Mirelle Vraimont is an internationally renowned concert singer who has had to manage food sensitivities on three continents. Food allergies, food sensitivities, weather condition management, variety in mold field management, etc., caused her to compile a series of techniques whereby one can manage one's own allergies and sensitivities, thereby, controlling health and weight. With a limited wardrobe needed in some of the hotter climates, she had to be sure that she could fit into the prescribed concert attire from Paris to New York to Porto Alegre (Brazil) to Joao Pessoa (Brazil).

In addition to her concert career and international travels, she is a published author, philosopher, and poet; teacher, parent, and patent holder. She traveled to more than fifteen different countries and has had the opportunity to observe firsthand the foods of the world, and through trial and error, determined the foods she could and could not use. As a vegetarian, she knows the complexity of finding foods that are tasty, beautiful to present, nutritious, health/life giving, and yet within the confines of her personal predilections.

She has raised three healthy and successful children and offers information to them yearly about the protections afforded by correct diet, dietary supplements, herbal supplements, exercise, healthy food preparation, homeopathic medicines, and quality living. It is her firm belief that vitamins are "insurance" and that taking them can only enhance one's health and well being. Remember the old adage: "If it can't help me, it certainly won't harm me."

It became clear to her that one can only manage one's *own weight*. We have certain foods that we prefer. Each of us guards his/her own health and are in absolute control of food intake, medical treatments, managing differing and difficult environments, health, and quality of life. We can and must take responsibility for our own weight.

It is hoped that by presenting this information and showing the absolute control one has over one's health primarily by what one eats that her fellow Americans will take control of their own health, weight, and well being, and come to the realization that with their own personal choices in the areas of food selection, exercise, vitamin supplementation, managing their daily intake, self-limiting strategies, and lifestyle choices, they can come to their ideal weight and remain there for a lifetime with a little self-discipline. They can also take their children along because if they offer the best food that can be found on the planet, the children will have formed personal predilections for fresh, life-giving, healthful foods, and most of the "junk" will remain just that: "junk."

Made in United States
Troutdale, OR
11/03/2026

56844364R00073